The Trouble with Therapy

The Trouble with Therapy
Sociology and Psychotherapy

PETER MORRALL

Open University Press

Open University Press
McGraw-Hill Education
McGraw-Hill House
Shoppenhangers Road
Maidenhead
Berkshire
England
SL6 2QL

email: enquiries@openup.co.uk
world wide web: www.openup.co.uk

and Two Penn Plaza, New York, NY 10121–2289, USA

First published 2008

A catalogue record of this book is available from the British Library

ISBN–13: 9780335218752 (pb) 9780335218769 (hb)
ISBN–10: 033521875X (pb) 0335218768 (hb)

Library of Congress Cataloging-in-Publication Data
CIP data applied for

Typeset by YHT Ltd, London
Printed in the UK by Bell and Bain Ltd, Glasgow

Fictitious names of companies, products, people, characters and/or data that may be used herein (in case studies or in examples) are not intended to represent any real individual, company, product or event.

The **McGraw·Hill** Companies

For dear Heather

Contents

Acknowledgements

While labouring on this book I have been very grateful for advertent and inadvertent enlightenment about therapy from the following friends, colleagues, and therapists (in alphabetical order): Dr John Adams; Jenny Archard; Jackie Ferguson; Dr Gina Glouberman; Professor Mike Hazelton; Ted Killan; Kirsty Kurtis; Barbara Kyle; Dr Paul Marshall; Dr Sue Pattison; Pauline Philips; Gordon Teal; Dr Nick Thyer; Dr Jenny Waite-Jones; Dr Jane Walford.

In all probability most of the above, if not all, do not agree with much, if any, of the content.

A very special thank you goes to Len and, of course, dear Heather.

Introduction

Trouble
Sceptic
Heather

This is a book about therapy[1] and sociology. It is also about a very special 'client', Heather. But, before introducing Heather, let me introduce the rationale for the book.

Trouble

I'm a trouble-maker. It is difficult for me not to be so. Possibly this is a trait spawned from a mutated bit of DNA, an evolutionary quirk that is functional to my genetic survival (but not necessarily that of all humankind), or an unconscious defence mechanism protecting me from realizing my

psychological failings. More likely, it is an adaptation learned from prolonged (nearly 30 years) exposure to sociology.

Sociology has built its reputation on causing trouble. In doing so
attracted much hostility, being critical about lots of people (politicians,
priests, and the police) and lots of things (capitalism, communism, liberalism, love, marriage, and McDonald's). Sociologists are socialized into
being troublesome: asking lots of challenging questions about what are
otherwise taken-for-granted ideas, values and social edifices. In doing so,
sociologists antagonize those with vested interests in what has become
accepted as the true and moral (the power elites), and those who just don't
want to bother contemplating such things (the intellectually indolent).

My career in being troublesome with respect to therapy began many
years ago for me when I attended a therapy 'summer school' to learn, over a
period of five days, how to be a therapist. This was in the days long before
regularization and certification, and prior to the legitimatization of the
'quickie therapy' (that is, the quick-to-learn and to quick-to-deliver variations of cognitive behavioural therapy).

The designer of the model, who was a major therapy guru at the time,
was always in attendance. He gave a hallowed homily early each morning in
which he described the segment of the model to be practised that day by the
participants (that is, the consumers of this particular therapeutic commodity). Skills practice was under the vigilant guidance of a group of
trainers. These trainers formed a quasi-military squad of pre-emptive
interventionists long before anyone had heard of neo-conservative policies.
Instruction was first through 'fish-bowl' demonstrations by the trainers, and
then intimidating close-quarter supervision of role-play by the participants
(the one who took the role of client was obliged to use 'real' issues). So, the
stock phrases, intonations, and actions of each bit of the model were learned
bit by bit, until lo and behold, a week later, the participant could put all the
bits together and solve *any* problem (whether this was his/her own or of that
of a client, and whether it was personal, mechanical, or ethereal).

The squad had its own hierarchy and highly specialized division of
labour. It was commanded by the astute if scary organizer of the summer
school (the 'General'). Below her were 'consultants' (the officers). Underneath the consultants were the instructors (the non-commissioned officers),
and, finally, the neophyte instructors (the 'poor bloody infantry'). Selection
into the squad, and movement up the ranks, were mainly through a mixture
of aptitude, nepotism, availability, and, for the 'poor bloody infantry', a
willingness to do most of the work for no pay. For the military analogy to
work in Britain, the guru would have been the Queen (no offence intended
to either party).

The regimented method of learning at this summer school was labelled as 'therapy by numbers' by my then highly cynical partner, herself a trained therapist. My ex-partner, was, it turned out, also highly cynical about me. But, I'm not bitter. Rather, I'm grateful for her (sociological) insight into the absurdly constricted and naïve nature of therapy. Some 20 years later, what is still the situation in therapy (certainly for most basic courses), is a reckless lack of concern about (global) society. In order to gain the required 'in-house' knowledge, skills, and attitudes (the supposed qualities of the 'good therapist'), there is either little time and scant motivation to persuade students to raise their gaze from their own navels and see the 'bigger picture' of world events concerning human suffering.

At the very first summer school there was a little trouble. A handful of unruly participants (including myself), drunk on bar talk (or just drunk) decided to defy the aura of conformity instilled by the squad. We, much to the explicit and fervent disapproval of some of the officer-consultants, formed a seditious discussion group to talk about why therapy seemed to ignore society, and social factors such as the skewed social profile of the hundreds of people at the conference. Out of the hundreds of people at the summer school that first year, none appeared to be from any ethnic minority group, and most seemed to be middle class. There were a few rough diamonds, working-class, hard-driven individuals (ex-nurses, and secretaries), and one or two people from the ranks of the unemployed. But these people were training in therapy trade to improve their occupational status, an example of *embourgeoisement* (the working classes aspiring to a middle-class lifestyle). This was 1980s Britain, the era of Thatcherism. Prime Minister Margaret Thatcher, somewhat disingenuously, was reported as saying that 'society didn't exist'. Her government's political philosophy owed much to the monetarist and libertarian views of US economist Milton Friedman. Government involvement in social welfare and as the employer of millions was to be reduced. Restrictions on industry and employment practices were to be removed, and the big trade unions smashed. Thatcher wanted a resurgence of small-scale businesses. Hence, setting up private therapy practice fitted in with the political and economic ideology of the day.

In this climate, our summer school *putsch*, like the rebellion of the teachers and miners before us, failed. After an altercation (in the bar) between the rebels and a particularly demonstrative consultant, the will to fight the governing class fizzled out.

We then knuckled down to become experts in the art of 'therapy by numbers'.[2] But worse, to my eternal shame, I was to betray the spirit of the revolution among the more socially aware summer school participants. I joined 'the squad'.

Despite very little therapeutic talent, but with favourable connections, I eventually became not just a neophyte but a *proper* instructor. Moreover, after a series of these summer schools I began to inflict my robotic model of therapy on actual clients. But my therapy career was short-lived. This was for two very good reasons: first, I never became good at it; second, my trouble-making career went in other directions (madness and murder), before returning to looking at therapy with the troublesome imagination of a sociologist.

Jeffrey Masson is another trouble-maker. I'm assuming that Masson, like me, is content to be so described. In the Foreword to Masson's seminally trouble-making book *Against Therapy*, the renowned therapist and author Dorothy Rowe wrote, presumably with Masson's agreement: 'Jeffrey Masson is a trouble maker. Every one of his books has been written to create trouble' (Rowe, in Masson 1990: 7). I don't know Masson personally. Nor do I agree whole-heartedly with his published views (I am not *against* therapy). But what I do know is that his contentions have incited 'thinking' (and probably a great deal of anger). That is my intention – to provoke reflection by those *in* the 'therapeutic enterprise' or who are reflecting *on* the therapeutic enterprise. By therapeutic enterprise, I am referring to the elements of therapy (the therapists, their habits, their organizations, and the stack of 'stuff' that therapy generates).

Aside from wishing to contribute to the understanding of the nature of therapy because of my sociological inheritance and dalliance with the practice of therapy, I have wanted to do so for some considerable time because of other relevant experiences. I used to believe that I had a rather exceptional if stigmatized relationship career. By 40 years of age I had been married and divorced twice, and indulged in serial monogamy whenever the opportunity arose. But this relationship pattern isn't so unusual today in the West. About 50 per cent of marriages end in divorce, and having multiple partners during one's lifetime, which could stretch to 80 years, is now unexceptional. Such a trend in relationships brings many people into contact with relationship 'helpers' of one sort or another. Indeed, I have been a client of one such relationship service.

Relate (2008) is Britain's largest provider of relationship counselling (as well as sex therapy). It has more than 600 centres for face-to-face therapy, a telephone service, and an internet facility. It is non-profit-making, but normally a fee is charged for face-to-face sessions (although this may be subsidized by the organization). Some counsellors working under licence for *Relate* operate as private practitioners and set their own fees. In 2008, the costs for using *Relate* were £45 (US$22.5) per hour on the telephone; and each reply from a counsellor by email £28.50 (US$14).

Each year *Relate* deals with about 150,000 clients. That's an awful lot of unhappy relationships. Moreover, although *Relate* is the key relationship-repairing establishment in Britain, there are many other organizations dealing with thousands of clients each year. Then there are the people, perhaps the majority of those in a relationship, who have problems with their partners at some time or another but who do not seek help from professional helpers. Misery in human interactions is hardly pathological if it is so common (which again, for a self-confessed relationship-bodger like me, is rather comforting).

My encounter with *Relate* was, I hope, idiosyncratic. There were, however, two idiosyncratic events. The first was a therapy session early in the process of trying to sort out the mess my (ex-)wife and I had got ourselves into. After two sessions with our therapist, it was decided by the counsellor that she needed to see us separately in order to understand, she explained, our personal histories prior to the marriage. When my turn came I dredged up harrowing tales from my childhood and embarrassing disclosures about my sexual awakenings, along with any other irksome event in my life I thought might be of interest to someone trying to figure out why I was the way I was. There was an hour and a half of interrogation and confession which left me emotionally exhausted. But, at no subsequent session with the therapist were any of my excavated ordeals and declared deviances referred to openly or implicitly. This left me wondering what the point was of the detailed raking over the past. I remain to this day mystified.

The second peculiar incident followed six 'free' sessions with this therapist. My then spouse and I agreed (a highly remarkable achievement) to employ a *Relate* therapist privately, who would visit us in our home. Everything went as could be predicted for the first three sessions (lots of bickering). Then during the fourth session, the therapist, quite reasonably, suggested that we should decide to either resolve the squabbling or dissolve the marriage. Well, I don't know what happened to the counsellor, but when the time came for the fifth session she didn't turn up, didn't send a message to explain why, and like some fly-by-night plumber who promised faithfully to fix a leaking pipe, was never seen again. To this day I am mystified about this as well.

But I'm not just a trouble-maker: I'm an angry trouble-maker.

The physical world is deteriorating, global society is in disarray, and humanity debased. Sociologists *and* therapists have a social responsibility to rage against such a mess. The existence of this mess *and* the lack of radicalism in the social sciences (which includes sociology, psychology, and therapy) make me *very* angry. This is not anger for which I need a therapist to help me 'come to terms with', displace, or sublimate. I *want* my anger. It is, for me, an affirming not a destructive emotion. I wish more of my fellow social scientists possessed such anger *and* that this anger would promote productive activism aimed at tackling the mess. Not to feel rage and enact this rage is both immoral and irrational. Therapy and sociology should be in the business not only of understanding humans and societies and/or of repairing individual lives, but also of working dynamically in the production and implementation of radical social policies. Too much time and energy is spent on the minutiae of institutional and personal agendas, rather than on what really matters. What really matters is tackling directly and virulently human suffering and social injustice *globally*.

Wealth, health, order, sanitation, and longevity co-exist with poverty, disease, disorder, violence, pollution, and death. Moreover, all of this deterioration, disorder, and debasement is the backdrop to the 'commodification' (an ugly piece of sociological jargon) of everything, including sex, death, walking, and (to use a much less ugly phrase by Thomas Szasz 1974) 'problems with living'. The enterprise of therapy is a, perhaps *the*, major stakeholder in the global commodification of problems with living.

Sceptic

But what causes this mess? The late Tony Banks, a former British Member of Parliament, blamed 'the horribleness of humanity'. He replied when asked the question by a journalist, 'What has been your most valuable life lesson?':

> This is easy. How vile human beings are as a species. If you look around at the enormous suffering that human beings inflict upon themselves, on other species and on the planet generally, you've got to come to the conclusion that, somewhere, nature went wrong. No doubt she will correct her error in due course.
>
> (Banks 2004)

I do not go as far as Banks in his cynical appraisal of humanity. There is much that humans should be proud about. I'd like to thank the Romans for inventing central heating (although with global warming affecting northern Europe, this may become a superfluous accomplishment). But, although the Romans brought central heating to Britain more than two thousand years previously, it has not as yet been installed in the cold and damp house. So, a second thank you from me goes to Sir Alexander Fleming, the Scottish biologist and Nobel Prize winner who serendipitously commenced the medical use of antibiotics. Without his luck and subsequent scientific skill, I would not have lived past childhood due to episodes of pneumonia (or so my mother believes).

Nor, as Banks implies, do I believe that humanity should wait for nature to correct the excesses and malevolence of humans. That might necessitate the wiping-out of humanity. Humans can replace devastation with preservation. Moreover, humanity may be stuck in state of *social atavism* (that is, at a point in the evolution of human civilization in which crime, violence, materialism, death and destruction are as apparent as altruism, love, spirituality, peace and harmony: Morrall 2006a). But they no longer live in caves (apart from fugitive terrorists and experimental anthropologists). Nor is it morally acceptable to bash over the head and drag off would-be mates (not even among the modern-day barbarian binge-drinking sexual predators – male and female – who invade British cities at weekends and European holiday resorts).

It is the role, not of cynic but of sceptic, that I adopt. With due respect to Banks, who did work tirelessly to improve the community he represented and died far too young, the cynic's contribution to society is usually one of pessimistic negativity. The sceptic's aim is not at all to be destructive. First, the sceptic takes the trouble (and in doing so can, of course, *cause* trouble) to examine propositions no matter who makes them. That is, nobody should be immune from such examination, whether he/she is Pope, President, professor, or therapy guru. Second, as Wendy Grossman (2006), editor of *The Skeptic* magazine points out, to be sceptical is not to destroy but to search for the evidence for any claim on truth, whether this is about alternative medicine, religion, creationism, superstring theory, sociology, psychology, or therapy.

Third, in my view, but not that of Grossman, the evidence sought by the sceptic does not need to be scientific. Indeed, I argue science itself should be viewed sceptically. Scientific endeavour may be fallible, but some reasoned justification, either in the form of well-developed theory and/or substantive empirical data, is expected before the sceptic can accept a proposition as 'true'. Furthermore, the sceptic accepts that 'truth' and 'reason' could be displaced by a new 'fact' or epistemology. Fourth, the task of the sceptic is to challenge the strength of a proposition, and if it is resolute, that's the job done. If not, then rather than leave ideas and practices 'deconstructed', the sceptic's job is to provide renovations or substitutes. Trouble-making and anger should have the ultimate goal of re-building even if some initial demolishing has to take place.

So, my roles as former therapist (unqualified and inexperienced), periodic client (eminently qualified and experienced), and *angry* sceptic (qualification and experience work in progress), have provided me with the impetus to write this book (which, of course, becomes another commodity in the therapy marketplace). The sociological critique presented here has the express aim of informing psychotherapy practice, and 'politicizing' that practice by examining and synthesizing its effects on people and society. It is placing sociology 'in' therapy *and* offering a sociology 'of' psychotherapy.

I am '*for* therapy'. Or rather I am for an *enlightened* therapeutic enterprise. The book begins with tools for enlightenment from the troublesome and sceptical trade of sociology which are applied throughout. These are four core sociological theories: structuralism; interactionism; constructionism (including postmodernism); and realism. As it stands, therapy is a 'Dr Jekyll and Mr Hyde' social institution, having some positive but many negative qualities. Specifically, *j'accuse* therapy of being: dysfunctional; arrogant; selfish; abusive; infectious; insane; and deceitful.

The depiction of the therapeutic enterprise as a unified and beneficent social institution, peopled by caring and empathic therapists working tirelessly and collectively for the good of their clients, is contested in Chapter 2. Therapy enterprise has a long history of conflicts and rivalries which remain today, and choosing a type of therapy and a therapist is a lottery. Therefore, the claim is made that therapy is a deeply dysfunctional discipline.

In Chapter 3, I suggest the therapeutic enterprise has become arrogant about efficacy. Therapy is being steadily legitimized through the application of science. That is, there has been a 'scientization' of therapy. But science is a conceited discourse (and by association, so is therapy). Apart from serious flaws in the politics and procedures of science, the scientific fallacy is that reality can be explained.

Chapter 4 explores the selfishness of therapy, that is, its overwhelming focus on the 'self'. The 'selfish' assumptions of therapy are challenged by examining external influences on human performance, and individualism (the idea that there are unitary and delimited 'individuals') is questioned. A sociological version of the self is then explored. The 'reflexive' self is one that interacts with society, with each affecting the other. However, the self is in danger of becoming saturated and thereby destroyed. Certainly, the self, in part because of the torrent of interest in sex from therapy, has become sodden with sexuality.

Chapter 5 considers how the enterprise of therapy is abusive. Personal power and social power are discussed. How power is structured and dispersed in society, to either empower or disempower individuals and social groups, is reviewed. Control in society and therapy, and the social role of therapy in the management of sickness, are evaluated.

In Chapter 6, the metaphor of 'infection' is applied to therapy. The therapeutic enterprise has embarked on a quest to make therapy a profession akin to medicine. But, too much therapy runs the risk of becoming poisonous in a similar way that 'medicalization' has become disabling. That is, 'therapyitis' (Morrall 2007b) undermines the individual's ability to take care of his/her own problems of living, and makes society dependent on therapists to sort out social problems.

The allegation made in Chapter 7 is that therapy is not only uninformed about global society, dysfunctional, arrogant, abusive, selfish, infectious, but also ignorant about its own business. Its business is madness. Although steeped in the tradition of medical understandings concerning human performance, the therapeutic enterprise displays limited awareness of the social history of psychiatry and the medicalization of madness. It has virtually no knowledge of how society impinges on sanity. These symptoms indicate that the institution of therapy should be certified as insane.

The final arraignment against the therapeutic enterprise, made in Chapter 8 is that therapy is deceitful. Therapy claims happiness is possible, and wants clients to be happy (or at least happier). There is a proliferation of 'positiveness' permeating therapy from psychology, providing all manner of reasons to be cheerful and recipes for rapture. However, the existence of inequality, disease, pollution, and violence indicates that nirvana and Shangri-La are illusory, and that the reality of the human condition and global society is not happiness but misery.

The Conclusion summarizes the trouble with therapy: dysfunction, arrogance, selfishness, abusiveness, infectiousness, insanity, and deceit, characterize the therapeutic enterprise. But therapy is not beyond redemption. Both the genuine magnanimity of therapists and the radical potential of the therapeutic enterprise are acknowledged. The suggestion is made that sociological enlightenment can be incorporated into the therapeutic enterprise (and it is recognized that there is an equivalent task for a trouble-making sceptical therapist to enlighten sociology). This could lead to sociology and therapy uniting and collaborating with other groups to tackle the reality of misery in global society by fermenting as much trouble as possible. Finally, the story of Heather reaches *its* conclusion.

Heather

Let me present Heather properly. Heather makes regular appearances in the book to help illustrate points being made in each chapter about therapy and the application of sociology to therapy.

Heather is a real person. There are some clarifications, however, about her realness: the story of Heather was told to me second-hand; a few details have been modified in order to ensure her anonymity and of those in her story; Heather, as with all of us, is not 'one person' – her 'self' has many compartments and the version(s) here presented will offer an interpretation which Heather would probably not recognize to be her real self.

Heather has troubles. Heather's troubles are intractable, numerous, and multilayered. But Heather is not an atypical human. She is not from Mars or Venus. Nor is she a caricature. Rather, she is a *characterization* of humanness. She represents what is present in all of us and contemporary society: intricacy and inconsistency. Just how much human intricacy and inconsistency is related to the intricacies and inconsistencies of contemporary global society is questioned in this book, as is the role of therapy in dealing with human and social dilemmas.

Heather is strikingly attractive, statuesque, green-eyed, greying-blonde, and with a body shape to suit her middle years (previously toned parts now noticeably rounded, but still short of chubby). Think of Major 'Hot Lips Houlihan', the head-nurse in the 1970s–1980s television series *M*A*S*H*. Captain Hawkeye Pearce said of Hotlips Houlihan, 'the woman is a paradox' (Series 1), and Major Charles Emerson Winchester III described her as 'a cross between seductress and Attila the Hun' (Series 6). Both men were bewildered and beguiled by Houlihan in equal measure.

Heather has an acute intelligence and precise articulation, and a penetrating and adroit wit which she often displays through insightful observations or adroit wordplay. But, Heather is at times also contemptuous, intemperate, and insensitive. She can cut 'down to size' any perceived adversary with a knock-out verbal blow. However, her destructive tendency frequently turns inwards. She is a 'psychological suicide bomber', injurious to others and to her own well-being.

From her first marriage to 'Saint', Heather has two young children, identical twins Bob and Bert. Saint, a skilled artisan, is so called because of his redoubtable decency, forbearance, serenity, and dedication to his children and the interests of others: a veritable male Mother Teresa. Heather and her current husband Damian (an estate agent[3] who has the demeanour of, and the desire to be, a social worker) have a ground-floor garden apartment within a large Georgian house in a fashionable south-east of England city. Heather and Saint share the parenting of Bob and Bert equally, although their legal residence is with their father.

As a mature student Heather gained a first-class degree in English and French at her local and highly prestigious university. She then excelled in the practical side of a teacher's training course, and accepted an appointment as a primary school-teacher. Heather has had a number of other jobs, including working as a solicitor's 'runner' (doing menial errands for a local law firm) until asked to leave when her then boyfriend was convicted of 'doing a runner' with other people's belongings.

Heather and her mother, a retired nursing sister with a tolerant and pleasant disposition, who is always prepared to do a simple kindness, have a strong bond. But Heather has had a markedly ambivalent relationship with her father, from childhood and throughout adulthood. She loves him for his generosity, and respects him for his practical abilities. But she also regards him as unemotional, uncommunicative, and authoritarian. All of her life she craved the sort of attention from him which he appeared so willing to give her older brother. Although she received his discipline and direction, she believes she has had to fight persistently for his love and approval (a battle she suspects she can never win).

At school, Heather, although patently academically capable and a gifted musician, never reached her full potential. Throughout adult life Heather, because of her good looks, has attracted attention from men (and a number of women). Heather is capable of giving fervent affection (particularly to her children), but she finds sexual expressiveness and mutuality difficult. Moreover, her sexual orientation is ambiguous.

Heather also fluctuates between behaving condescendingly, egoistically, offensively, or childishly, when trying to get her own way, and taking charge effectively and efficiently of demanding situations. She also vacillates between tolerance and bigotry, astuteness and obtuseness, compassion and meanness, timidity and assertiveness, ruefulness and ruthlessness, and victim and victimizer. Moreover, although Heather is adamant that she hasn't a 'maternal instinct', she does have exemplary parental skills.

Certain situations Heather finds stressful and she will make strenuous efforts to circumvent – whenever her honesty, loyalty or capability is in doubt. At such times she has been know to fugue (a psychiatric term meaning either to literally run away or to emotionally switch off). If she is unable to get away, she becomes belligerent. But, she will also defend fearlessly and befriend sincerely the socially disadvantaged and demonized.

Perfectionism is a noticeable trait in Heather, although sometimes this is disguised as avoidance or indolence. That is, Heather will only tackle any activity (cerebral or physical) if she considers that she will do it flawlessly. Whether it's cleaning her home, sitting examinations, playing the piano, singing the blues, or 'arm-rustling',[4] she must be the best. Otherwise, she will not take the risk of doing anything that she might not reach her own high standard. Being second is not an option, but opting out is.

So, Heather has psychological dissonance – the noble and the ignoble parts of her 'self' collide. She is pathologically insecure and has an abject terror of rejection. Moreover, Heather's 'Dr Jekyll and Mr Hyde' persona, while it can be found in everyone to a greater of lesser extent, is amplified in her. She seems unable or unwilling to settle on being either an angel or devil, and bounces between the two much more starkly than most people. If anyone could benefit from therapy (and that assumption is questioned in this book), then it is this indubitably troubled yet indisputably fascinating woman.

Heather has tried therapy. Over a five-year period she attended a few sessions with formally trained therapists. But she also received prolonged informal therapy, both solicited and unsolicited, from Len.

Len, a journalist, having had a basic (unregulated and uncertificated) training in the art of lively listening and compassionate confrontation to assist in the interviewing he conducts for his work, became Heather's well-meaning but ultimately inept 'barefoot therapist' during their passionate, turbulent, and doomed relationship. His munificent but misguided intention was to enlighten Heather. 'Len' is a pseudonym chosen by me because of his propensity to misappropriate and macerate the words of his artistic hero, the poet, songwriter, and connoisseur of gloom, Leonard Cohen. Len is the primary informant for Heather's story.

Enlightenment

Imagination

Structuralism

Interactionism

Constructionism

Realism

Chapter 1 is about the enlightening theories of sociology. But mere mention of this 'ology' is enough to make membership of the Plain English Society increase meteorically. An unbridled fear of suffocation from a blanket of jargon might not be unusual in the uninitiated, but even students of sociology groan involuntarily at the prospect of grappling with 'theory'. Certainly, Heather, who had to study the subject as part of her university education, loathes what she considers as the pretentiousness of sociologists. She especially detests their (alleged) convoluted and extravagant linguistic ramblings, for which she uses a rather unpleasant (and physically unfeasible) description. Heather's estimation of therapy is no less iconoclastic.

However, while I am mindful of the impenetrability of some sociological concepts, there is also a necessity for tenacity and diligence to appreciate any academic subject. These traits are in their infancy in Heather, and are anyway not very conducive to a fast-moving and information-overloaded electronic global society (Heather also abhors electronic 'gadgets', computers, the internet, and email). But ideas generated from sociology and other academic subjects (including therapy), are by their very nature difficult and should not be abridged merely because they need more attention than television soap operas or the lyrics of popular music. Lucid language should be a goal in communication, but simplifying complex thinking can result in a loss of meaning, which can then only be regained by working backwards to increase the level of sophistication, making the exercise pointless.

Apart from the problem of 'jargon', sociology has a conceptualization of human performance (behaviour, thinking, and emotions[1]) which usually differs from that of therapy, but also can give the impression of being somehow superior. As part of my initiation into the subject when I started my undergraduate degree, one respected but aloof lecturer declared to the class that sociologists are 'different'. Looking around the classroom, filled as it was with a motley mix of embarrassingly eager mature students, deflated teenagers who had been rejected from more prestigious institutions, proto-revolutionaries, 'young liberals' (there was such a political sect at this time), and the politically flaccid, along with a few who seemed to have been transported from distant lands (finding themselves on this course if not by mistake then without due care and attention to their educational aspirations), my immediate thought was that he had a point. But I'd misjudged him. What he was really implying was that the 'professional' (deemed so from day one of the course) study of society fomented a uniquely sophisticated view of everything in society and about all societies. We, a disparate amalgam of talents and tendencies, were special!

It may seem elitist or delusional to suggest that there is something exceptional about the way in which sociologists view humans and the world they inhabit. Certainly, sociology (usually) offers different understandings from those arising from other academic disciplines such as psychology and biology (given that sociology, as with psychotherapy and biology, does not have a fully unified epistemology[2]).

In this chapter 'the sociological imagination' (that is, the 'specialness' of sociology) is delineated through an exploration of four key theoretical frameworks. I am using the phrase 'theoretical framework' to describe the grouping of ideas that can be brought together to support a bigger idea (for example, a number of ideas about how the universe began – gravity, relativity, Big Bang, and superstrings – have been assembled under the theoretical framework of 'M-theory'). Theoretical frameworks with similar philosophical routes, and complementary methods to substantiate a bigger idea (for example, the bringing together of the laws of physics, chemistry, mathematics, and cosmology under 'science') form an 'epistemology'. Epistemology, therefore, means a collection of theoretical frameworks that define a particular type of knowledge.

The first theoretical framework I have chosen regards society as both existing and having a set of configurations that to a greater or lesser extent induce humans to perform in pre-ordained ways. Moreover, these influences on human performance can be discovered through (social) scientific method. The *structuralist* understanding of human performance, in its extreme, views all behaviours, thoughts, and emotions as 'determined' by society. Human performance (especially changing misery to happiness) can be manipulated through social engineering rather than therapeutic enlightenment. Therefore therapy for the structuralist may be either pointless or counterproductive, part of the problem rather than the solution, if personal and social ills are bred by how society is organized.

But the second explanatory genre is more sympathetic to the notion of individual volition. The *interactionist* position is that, while there are structures in society, humans can and do give 'meaning' to their own lives, and that allows them to transgress the boundaries of these structures. Interactionism hence can find commonality with some types of therapy, that is those that do deliberate over the influence of social 'systems' (the wider and multifarious networks of contacts humans have with others, for example, through family ties, work, leisure activities, and mass electronic communications).

The *constructionist* position, which is the third theoretical framework, takes the interactionist stance further by positing that 'reality' is not what it seems, and can be 'deconstructed'. At its (postmodernist) extreme, all human performance, all social entities, all physical matter, and all scientific laws, are considered as merely accepted 'constructs'. Some therapists have gone the postmodernist way, offering their clients the possibility of manufacturing their very own epistemology (that is, a view of the world that *they* can decide works for them).

Fourth is the perspective of *realism*. Realism is an amalgam of structuralism and interactionism/constructionism. There is for the realist an acceptance of 'facts' (social and natural reality), but these facts are obscured by cultural meanings. Moreover, extant epistemologies and their associated modes of investigation (science and the scientific method) have so far proven to be inadequate in finding and therefore explaining reality.

Imagination

> To understand the changes of many personal milieux we are required
> to look beyond them ... To be able to do that is to possess the
> sociological imagination.
>
> (Mills 1959: 10/11)

Humans have, since the first collections of hominoids in the African rain-
forests tens of millions of years ago, existed within social milieux. That is,
they virtually always belong to social groupings of one type or another.
Humans for thousands of years have belonged to multiple social groupings,
their families, and then at least one layer of social assemblage beyond that
of the family.

Today, this social milieux includes multiple varieties of the family (for
example, single parent; nuclear; polygamous; extended; step; and gay/
lesbian), various associations, sub-cultures, and communities (based on, for
example, religion; volunteer work; pastimes; or deviancy), society (the
nation or supra-nation), global society, and cyberspace. The exceptions
might be hermits or castaways, although even they have come from and
may go back to their social groups.

Private troubles – public issues

The sociologist, therefore, considers seemingly exclusively personal states
such as happiness, misery, hate, envy, shyness, erotic arousal, mental disorder, contentment, and empowerment to be linked inexorably to social
factors. It was C. Wright Mills (1959) who pointed to the connection
between 'private troubles' and 'public issues'. Whatever we do as individuals (what we feel, how we act, and what we think), it has some
connection with our social surroundings.

For example, the private trouble of losing a loved one in a car accident is
a public issue in that both the amount of money governments put into road
safety, and the degree to which a society values commodities such as cars,
are linked to the number of people who are killed on the roads. The private
trouble of being diagnosed as having cancer is also a public issue as either
directly or indirectly it relates to health policy and health service resources,
which in turn are connected to economic policies and political decisions.
Better health promotion strategies installed by government and health
agencies, a greater political will at a local and national level to improve the
physical environment, more money ploughed into cancer research and
treatment rather than, for example, conducting warfare, might have pre-
vented that person's malignant tumour. The private trouble of depression is

a public issue in the sense that this 'internal' condition may have been precipitated by alienating and dehumanizing social circumstances.

Even the private trouble of committing murder has social connotations. A society that revels in violence sets the stage for such seemingly volitional acts as taking, with malice aforethought, someone's life. Governments, criminal justice systems, mass media, authors, and sporting organizations orientate the individual's personal potential to kill. Declaring war, enacting the death penalty, producing horror films, writing about heinous events, and engaging in highly competitive contact games, while not necessarily directly the cause, provide the social atmosphere in which murder is not considered peculiar and perhaps fascinating (Morrall 2006a).

Heather's 'private troubles' have links to her family, and the social *milieux* in which she spent her childhood and schooling. Her feelings of insecurity and rejection, which furnished her sexual ambiguity, a need for control, drive for perfectionism, and aggression, are rooted in early socialization. In turn, this socialization was shaped by, for example, post-Second World War governmental educational and welfare policies, and the shifting social norms concerning the gender roles. As an adult, the interrelationship between Heather's troubles and society continued, but were different. For example, for women in the West, there had been a huge change in role expectation relating to education, employment, domesticity, child-rearing, sexuality, and partner selection. Heather's mother had already paved the way for Heather to be less hide-bound by convention. Having trained as a nurse before she was married, but stopped paid employment to rear Heather and her brother, she went back into nursing and has had a successful career. However, her father is of the 'old school' concerning what women should do, and her brother has been caught in his own socially generated issues of uncertainty about what role young men should play in society.

Asking 'why'

Social events and social relationships are not taken at face value by the sociologist. Moreover, sociology, despite what might be the public perception, is not merely common sense. At times, sociology coincides with conventional wisdom, but only after the veracity of the relevant assumptions has been tested through empirical research and/or systematic theorizing. At other times, what is ordinarily taken as fact is contradicted by sociological analysis.

The formal study of society was begun by August Comte (1798–1857) who, in 1838, conceived of the term 'sociology', and thereby inaugurated a new academic discipline. Many of Comte's ideas are to be found in the work of later theorists. The literal interpretation of the word 'sociology', coming from the Latin 'socius' and 'ology' is the study of companionship. A definition I have used is: 'Sociology is the rigorous investigation of social phenomena using systematic theorising and/or methodical research procedures' (Morrall 2001: 10).

It is the use of theories and research (which have been scrutinized through exacting peer review and debate) that separates 'common sense' from substantive knowledge. However, sociological insights that may arise outside of this academic process can still be credible. Social scientists such as Michel Foucault do not stick to the rules of investigation. Foucault was imaginative in the extreme, but not consistently orderly when conducting social scientific investigation, what he called his 'archaeology of knowledge' (Foucault 1969). Nevertheless Foucault has been extremely influential in fomenting the sociological imagination about public issues such as power, madness and sexuality.

George Ritzer (2006) suggests that 'social thinking' (that is, the employment of the sociological imagination) involves a more disciplined, broader, orderly and deliberate manner, and reference to thoughts of previous social thinkers, than ordinary thinking. Essentially, the basis of the 'sociological imagination' is to look beyond the obvious and minutiae, and to challenge pre-conceived ideas (including those of sociologists). Above all, it is to always ask the question 'why', and to keep on asking the question 'why', scrutinizing systematically all possible answers. But to be imaginative sociologically does not necessarily rest on the procurement of empirical and/or theoretical evidence (that is, 'scientific' knowledge). Other 'archaeologies of knowledge' are possible, even if we do not know what they are yet. Hence, I have amended my definition of sociology to: 'Sociology is the rigorous *questioning* of social phenomena.'

Therapists (most of them) are also interested in asking 'why'. They want to know, for example, why humans behave and think in self-destructive ways or why this client keeps repeating the same series of mistakes in her/his life. But some therapists balk at the very idea of asking 'why' (especially with their clients as by doing so the client may focus unfruitfully, in the view of the therapist, on past events which cannot be altered or that do not actually have any bearing on the client's present problems). However, therapy in essence is only interested in the narrow aspects of human performance. In the main, therapy reduces the question of 'why' to an individual's history and circumstances, or at best that of her/his family and other close social networks.

Therapy (and psychology), therefore, are 'reductionist'. For example, the fifth edition of Windy Dryden's best-selling *Handbook of Individual*

Therapy alludes to its coverage of 'social contexts' (Dryden 2007). However, not one of its 19 chapters has any profound analysis concerning the global mess of human suffering that arises from social and health inequalities, violence, and impending ecological catastrophe. Nor do any of its authors have any obvious sociologically-minded credentials or roles. It is this reductionism that *my* 'sociological imagination' rails against.

Structuralism

The most significant contribution to the systematic understanding of society is that of structuralism. Sociology could not have become an academic discipline without the insights that structuralism offers about how society operates above and beyond that of the individuals who make up that society. Most, if not all, other theories in sociology either owe their philosophical allegiance to structuralism or are competing with its persuasive premise. Without this perspective the notion that humans are not always, if ever, in charge of their own lives would not have been considered for academic investigation. This consideration has major implications for personal responsibility and the ability humans have to change their lives. It therefore challenges some of the core convictions of therapy.

The structuralist stance is that humans belong to social groups and that it is membership of these groups, to a greater or lesser degree, that dictates human performance. Specifically, the institutions of society (including those of education, criminal justice, the family, industry and commerce, media, health, and therapy), and the ways in which society is divided (principally by socio-economic class, gender, ethnicity, religion, age, and geography) set out the boundaries for human performance.

These pre-ordained patterns to society are maintained by various ideologies (economic, political, cultural, and religious). These ideologies are regularized belief systems that indoctrinate humans (or attempt to do so). Communism, Christian evangelism, and patriarchy are examples of doctrines that recommend, if not dictate, how people should think, behave and feel. For example, (in Western society) messages about self-responsibility, self-betterment, materialism, health improvement, and social hierarchies, are overtly and subtlety endorsed by a number of social institutions (such as government crime, health, and education departments; television and news conglomerates). These messages present a 'normative' set of values, which the 'good citizen' is expected (and may be forced) to follow. What is being communicated through a mixture of explicit and implicit, verbal, non-verbal, printed and electronic transmissions, are the rules for acceptable performance. Those who don't abide by the rules, if they are found out, are denounced as 'deviants' or 'anti-social', thereby attracting the social control mechanisms of approbation and punishment.

Psychological states for the structuralist, are socially contrived. How the individual thinks and feels about his/her life is related to the social conditions surrounding him/her (such as poverty, bigotry, inequality, violence, cruelty, wealth, rivalry, equality, compassion, collaboration, and spirituality). Optimism, fatalism, or contentment therefore are sensations generated by his/her significant others, working environment, neighbourhood, and government. The client's (and therapist's) cognition and emotion are framed by these external influences. An element of cognitive and emotional re-indoctrination is possible within a session (that is, the client and therapist become for a short while – 50 minutes! – a micro-society), but the effect can only be minimal and temporary. There are so many stronger and enduring effects at play than what the therapist can offer.

Certainly, it is possible that a different perspective may be excited, which then could change how the client behaves. However, unless the outside world has also been transformed to harmonize with the therapist-induced one, then therapy is mere emollient. The structure of the world *is* changing rapidly. But it is highly unlikely to be in a manner complementary to the agenda of a particular therapy session, or if it is, then the client and therapist are acquiescing to external pressures, not the other way around.

From this standpoint, Heather's troubles, being the product of society, are unalterable through therapy. Moreover, Heather suspects that therapy is an impotent façade. Although she succumbed to a few formal therapy sessions and years of informal therapy from barefoot Len, she says she would rather drink a bottle (or two) of red wine or eat a (very large) bar of high-cocoa chocolate to alleviate any particularly bothersome emotional problem.

Auguste Comte thought there were general laws of society in a similar way to those of the natural world and therefore these could be studied scientifically as causes and effect connections could be discovered. He also regarded society as analogous to the human body. All structures of society, like the structures of the human body (for example, the heart, liver, brain, and colon) are interlinked. Each structure of society, as with the body, was dependent on the other parts, and just as humans have evolved, so society progressed through its historical stages towards greater complexity and sophistication.

Comte was 'holistic' in his approach to sociology. Society, according to Comte, was made up of inter-relating parts, *and* was an entity beyond that of its parts. Each human is made up of billions of molecules, genes, and

DNA. But it is not possible to understand humans fully by examining them at the level of their constituent elements. Microscopic examination of tissues along with genetic mapping reveals much information about how humans operate, but not enough to comprehend the personality, physique, and temperament of an individual, let alone why there are differences between humans. Melody is not discernible from scanning the series of notes on a music sheet. Similarly, for Comte, an understanding of society cannot be achieved by focusing on the performance of humans as individuals, or by aggregating these performances. To use a term used in therapy, humans have a 'gestalt' form, and so does society.

Emile Durkheim

Emile Durkheim (1858–1917) developed Comte's work, and became the founder of *functionalist* sociology. Functionalism retains Comte's scientific, holistic and gestalt view of society. But in addition it perceives all social institutions as having a purpose which is beneficial for society. Social institutions adapt to new needs as society evolves. Families have the function of socializing children into the norms of society, but as these norms have altered, so does the composition of the family (which can be nuclear, extended, step, single, or gay/lesbian). Law enforcement agencies have the function of sustaining social stability. However, as new threats appear (for example, terrorism, sex tourism, and cyber-crime), or old ones are given greater attention (for example, race hate, noisy neighbours, and truancy), then powers of arrest fluctuate, as do the type and number of agencies employed by the state. Universities, formerly bastions of elitist wisdom, now attempt to provide work-orientated skills and 'applied' knowledge to meet the demands of an ever more complex division of labour and competitive global economy.

The social institution of therapy has the function of benefiting the individual by reducing personal despair. Society can also gain if the client returns to work and resumes family responsibilities. But how is therapy evolving?

For Durkheim, sociological research should seek out social facts, and use methods (specifically, the social survey) that can illuminate the structural impositions of society on human performance. Durkheim, like all structuralists, rejected the reductionist view that social acts (for example, getting married, being ill, working as a therapist) could be explained by reference to individual motivation.

A major contribution made by Durkheim to the stucturalist argument was his empirical study of suicide (Durkheim [1897] 1966). Comparing cross-societal rates of suicide, he claimed that the structure of society was crucial to decisions about taking one's life. Whilst he accepted that for some people there was individual choice, a state of 'normlessness' (Durkheim's term was 'anomie'), engendered by an absence of systems of social support and strong belief systems, increased the likelihood of suicide. In those countries where family and religion were important, then people had tangible norms to give their lives poignancy, shape, and direction.

Durkheim's proposition about the social nature of suicide has been criticized for taking official figures as reliable. It may be that very family-orientated and religious countries tend to obfuscate the facts about fatal self-harm (Pope 1976). Moreover, functionalism doesn't usually take into account features of social institutions that are not beneficial to society or benefit only a few. For example, families can be abusive, the police and the courts can be considered as serving the interests of the ruling elite, universities may be used to 'mop up' the unemployed, and therapy may be making the population dependent and impotent.

A further criticism of functionalism is that by explaining social institutions in terms of their consequences, it offers a circular ('teleological') description rather than a deep analysis. For example, if asked the question, 'Why are most therapists women?', a functionalist might answer, 'Women are most suited to the emotional work of therapy.' There is little appreciation of other factors that need to be examined, such as how is it that men seem not to engage in the same way with emotions as women? Another example of teleology would be if the answer to the question 'Why does therapy exist?' was 'Because people have problems that therapy can help resolve.' Again, this is an insufficient response as people have always had problems, so why did therapy come about in a particular epoch?, why did it take the form it did?, and does it really help resolve human problems?

Notwithstanding this inherent deficit in the functionalist reasoning, Durkheim's observation that social structure dramatically affects human performance is a momentous one. Moreover, it has resonance in today's world. Many communities throughout the world are experiencing anomie. Consequently, global structures, not human disposition, should be the therapeutic target. Individual despair is grounded not in individual dysfunction but social dysfunction. Perhaps, this is how therapy can evolve. That is, take on a greater moral function in a global society, transcending its functionality for individuals and providential outcome for society? That is, does the state of the world not necessitate a deliberate and progressive maturation of therapy towards social justice rather than just personal problems?

Karl Marx

The structuralism of Karl Marx (1818–1883) offers insights into the working of society that supersede the functionalism of Durkheim. Marx's theories, most of which are connected to his unique account of history (emphasizing the importance of the economy in shaping human performance), relate to his and that of his co-theorist and friend Friedrich Engels' (1820–1895) experiences of nineteenth-century European industrialization.

Marx's prediction that social progress would be obtained through the ascendancy of socialism and then communism has been discredited. The Communist bloc of Eastern Europe and the Soviet Union collapsed in 1991. By 2006, only the (communist) Republic of Cuba and the Democratic People's (communist) Republic of Korea remained loyal to the socially progressive politics of Marx; the (socialist) People's Republic of China, and the Socialist Republic of Vietnam have joined the (capitalist) World Trade Organization.

However, Marx's investigation of the intricacies, corruptions, and conflicts in capitalism remain highly relevant in the twenty-first century. Moreover, his understanding of the detrimental effects of capitalism on human psychology is still pertinent.

In his early publications Marx ([1844] 1959) argued that the way capitalist society was structured caused people to become 'alienated' from their own humanity. Work, for Marx, was essential to humans because it allowed individuals to express their creativity, and encouraged social cooperation. But the upshot of the capitalist way of work, observed Marx, was the denial or restriction of creativity, and the substitution of social cooperation with interpersonal rivalry and exploitation. As employees of capitalist enterprises, people were no longer in control of their work as they had been within an agricultural 'mode of production' (Marx's term for a particular type of economy). Families managing the land, artisans, or the self-employed operating small-scale commercial outlets, expressed their 'self' in what they produced, and what they produced was in the main delivered to the local population. The capitalism mode of production shattered the intimate connection people had with their work. Industrialization, urbanization, and the move to employment in large-scale industrial factories resulted in people becoming estranged from what they were producing, and a loss of job satisfaction. Work became not a rewarding activity, but toil for others in return for money. In Marxist terms, workers have become 'wage slaves'.

The epitome of alienated work in industrial settings was the twentieth-century car 'assembly line'. A worker would have one small task to perform repeatedly without any need to comprehend how this fitted into the overall car design. By the twenty-first century much of this repetitive and insentient labour was being conducted by machines. However, computers were also responsible for the growth in another form of alienated work. There has been a huge growth in the number of computer operatives who sit in large 'office warehouses' dealing with insurance, banking, travel, and telecommunications. For example, globally, tens of millions of people (one million in the UK alone) are employed in call centres. Such office warehouses are associated with very low job satisfaction and have a high turnover of staff (Giddens 2006). Work is closely supervised, with the use of electronic surveillance on the increase to provide details of every move and conversation of employees. Moreover, since the 1990s there has been a resurgence of the nineteenth-century 'sweatshop' in the developed, developing and under-developed parts of the world, particularly in garment manufacturing (Sweatshop Watch 2006). The modern sweatshop, like its historical forerunner, is characterized by low wages, debt bondage, overcrowded and unsafe conditions. Furthermore, industrializing countries with rapidly emerging economies (principally China and India), are re-creating the miserable, insecure, degrading, and abusive conditions that Engels described in 1845 in his study of the English working class (Engels 1999).

Marx in his later work, the seminal text *Das Kapital* ([1867] 1971) highlighted the connection between the economic 'base' of a society and what makes up the rest of society (its 'superstructure'). The economic base is made up of: (1) the particular mode of production (examples of which are: ancient; feudal; agrarian; capitalist); (2) the machinery and technology used in the production of goods and services (the 'means of production'); (3) and two groupings of people. These groupings consist of, on the one hand, the people who do the work, and on the other, those who force them to do so, or employ them. According to Marx, throughout history these two groups have been in tension with one another. In ancient society it was slaves against the free citizens, in medieval times it was feudal nobility against the serfs, and in the industrial age the proletariat (the working class) against the bourgeoisie (the middle class).

The superstructure of a society is all the other institutions (for example: the church; the family; health systems; education; criminal justice; politics; media; and therapy), and their concomitant belief and practices. That is, what people feel, do, and think, is inspired by the economic system. Hence, in therapy the backdrop to all communication is the values inherent in the mode of production in which the client and therapist operate. There are, therefore, no neutral zones in which therapy can take place. An underlying bias is always present although usually not recognized as such, as this bias would actually be regarded as the 'norm'.

Marx argued that it was the conflict between the 'exploited' and the 'exploiters' in each type of economic system that led to change. He anticipated that capitalism would eventually change, either through evolution or revolution (depending on which interpretation of Marx's writing is adopted), into an economic system without exploitation (that is, to a communist mode of production).

Exploitation occurs for Marx under capitalism through forcing people to work in dangerous and filthy surroundings in monotonous jobs, and with no power to influence the running of the factory or business. But his significant contribution to the study of economics was to identify how the bourgeoisie exploited the proletariat. He realized an employee may produce goods worth a certain amount when these goods are sold, but the employee received much less than that amount as wages. The rest, the 'surplus value', was the profit for the bourgeoisie.

Crucially, for Marx, the economic base directs the shape and denotation of everything else in society (that is, the superstructure). For Marx, the capitalist form of economy is supported by an ideology that favours the interests of the bourgeoisie (which for Marx in nineteenth-century Europe, was also the ruling class).

Marx thought that capitalism, like all other economic systems, would eventually collapse due to its 'internal contradictions'. The swings in employment/unemployment, the ultimate limit of available markets, the spread of wars to defend existing markets, and the increase in trade union activity collectivizing the demands of working peoples, would be the catalysts. However, far from a collapse of capitalism, there has been a globalization of capitalism. Capitalism in the twenty-first century is virtually pandemic. Globalization refers to the increasing economic, technological and cultural interdependence of humans living throughout the world in a 'global village' (McLuhan 1964; Giddens 2006).

Multinational capitalist businesses cut across national boundaries, and corporate power is challenging the authority of national politicians, with global (capitalist) financial organizations such as the World Bank and the International Monetary Fund instructing governments on fiscal management. As Hywel Williams (2006) comments, the politicians have little influence on national economies in the face of the power of the business and financial elites who do not owe allegiance to any one country.

The globalization of capitalism has been prompted and maintained through the dissemination of a virulent and highly politicized ideology (what Antonio Gramsci describes as 'hegemony': Gramsci 1971). Western-based (largely US) economic philosophies have spread commodity fetishism and the mystification of reality to nearly every country. In the 2000s, the US neo-conservative government of President George W. Bush, aided by the British New Labour government of Tony Blair and an assortment of smaller countries, instigated pre-emptive military intervention in Iraq and Afghanistan, aimed at stabilizing the world.

In Marxist terms, the globalization of capitalism can be viewed as 'cultural imperialism'. By 'cultural imperialism', I am referring to exporting Western values concerning, for example, material possessions, employment, and health, to societies with other cultural practices. Moreover, mass electronic communication systems and media, along with international tourism, serve to increase the rate and penetration of the Western practices into other cultures.

Moreover, there has not only been a globalization of Western culture, but also of Western inequalities (Glyn 2006). Wealth is not shared equally between the developed (Western), developing (transitional/emerging), and under-developed (stagnating/declining) countries of the world, or within these countries. The widening inter-societal and intra-societal inequality gap has produced a global elite, extracting surplus value from a globalized workforce. Both the elite and the workforce are increasingly itinerant, the former moving to areas of the world where trade can be conducted with minimal restrictions and costs, and the latter searching for employment wherever it can be found. In a hegemonized global village, the Chinese, Indian, Russian, and Brazilian bourgeoisie culturally have more in common with their counterparts in Europe, Australasia, and North America, than they do with their fellow non-elite citizens. Philippe Legrain (2006) argues that globalization is working. There has been a reduction in global inequality, he suggests. Most noticeably, China and India are catching up economically with the West, but so are a number of other Asian and South American countries. The exception is Sub-Saharan Africa, but for Legrain what it needs is more, not less, globalization to yank it out of poverty.

Western-orientated therapy is also being globalized. Therapy has been 'exported' to developing and under-developed countries, as part of this cultural imperialism. The use of therapy in developing and under-developed countries may be laudable. For example, it is hard to denounce therapy when it is directed towards helping people prevent or cope with HIV/AIDS, manage post-traumatic stress inflicted by warfare, or overcome the consequences of childhood abuse. However, from the Marxist viewpoint, it is part of a package of culturally-invasive aspirations that buttresses capitalism.

That Marx's ideas are still relevant to today's world was underscored in 2005 when he was chosen by listeners to the highbrow BBC Radio 4's *Today* programme as their favourite philosopher of all time. Furthermore, as Francis Wheen, author of the highly praised biography on Marx (Wheen 2000), observes:

> Fifteen years ago, after the collapse of communism in Eastern Europe, there appeared to be a general assumption that Marx was now an ex-parrot. He had kicked the bucket, shuffled off his mortal coil and been buried forever under the rubble of the Berlin Wall. No one need think about him – still less read him – ever again.

> 'What we are witnessing,' Francis Fukuyama proclaimed at the end of the Cold War, 'is not just the … passing of a particular period of postwar history, but the end of history as such: that is, the end point of mankind's ideological evolution.'

> But history soon returned with a vengeance. By August 1998, economic meltdown in Russia, currency collapses in Asia and market panic around the world prompted the *Financial Times* to wonder if we had moved 'from the triumph of global capitalism to its crisis in barely a decade'. The article was headlined 'Das Kapital Revisited'.

The Fukuyama thesis (Fukuyama 1993), referred to above by Wheen, was that the version of liberal-democratic capitalism championed by the USA had defeated all political, economic, and ideological challengers – forever. But some thirteen years later even Fukuyama can see the cracks in the otherwise triumphant capitalist mode of production, accepting that all is not going well with the end of history, given the neo-conservatives in the USA had not succeeded in their pre-emptive quests to stabilize the Middle East (Fukuyama 2006).

Structuralism has not been applied to therapy to any sweeping degree, but some feminist therapists have borrowed from the approach (Seu and Heenan 1998; Chaplin 1999). Insights into how the continued patriarchal structure of Western societies, and the embedded patriarchy of Islamic culture, inhibits the full emancipation of women at work, in politics, and in the home, are relevant considerations when trying to decipher why women view themselves in a particular way (Mirkin 1994; Seu and Heenan 1998; Chaplin 1999). It may be, for example, that the debilitating guilt Heather experienced following the birth of her children was stirred up by social pressure arising from an outdated perception of how a 'good mother' should feel. Heather realized that she did not have a 'maternal instinct'. However, although she received much social disapproval for not having this 'natural' female quality, far from being a 'bad mother', she excelled at parenting. That is, she and Saint carried out blended roles, mixtures of mother–father facets (with Heather giving more emphasis to fathering and Saint to mothering).

Interactionism

An alternative sociological approach to that of structuralism is interactionism. The interactionist position, as with much of psychology and therapy, is that humans give 'meaning' to their performance. Hence, the interactionist argument on first reading seems to be akin to most psychological theories (and therefore most therapy approaches) – but it is not.

Symbolic interactions

Interactionist sociology is not the same as psychology or therapy because social contexts are taken into consideration. That is, whatever and however humans perform, social factors will provide the background to, and hence some influence over, that performance. One way this happens is through 'symbolic interactions'. When humans communicate with each other, they give and receive messages about what is valued in that situation. These verbal and non-verbal symbols (for example, a head movement implying disagreement, an affirmative grunt, quizzical expression, or an angry outburst) give value and direction to the communications. This results in an ever-changing process of forming and re-forming what sense we make of our world, what is socially acceptable to others, what to think about our own thoughts, which emotions are appropriate generally or related to particular issues, and what our past actions connote and how we should act in the future. Interactions, therefore, shape what we come to understand as our 'self', and shape that understanding of 'self' in others. 'Self' is particularly susceptible to refashioning during therapy as this is a social context that is usually very symbolic. The client is frequently explicitly (if not always knowingly) attending therapy to alter aspects of his/her present self, the bits that are causing difficulties to him/her. Although perhaps to a lesser extent in the main than the client, the therapist is also changing through interactions with the client and systems of evaluation (either through the therapist's own reflections or through supervision).

Relevant social contexts of therapy sessions would include the training and perspective of the therapist, the social identity of the therapist and the client (such as age, gender, and ethnicity), and the contractual agreement made for the therapy. Society also provides wider contextual influences. For example, the social status of therapy, and legal and consumer rights for clients.

Moreover, the symbolic value of interactions within therapy will be affected by external social conditions. For example, when a therapist discusses with a client the latter's impending loss of employment, this will have a different symbolism if it is in a country which does not have the safety net of welfare provision for the unemployed compared with another country that does. If a female client's marriage is in disarray within a liberal democracy, where divorce and the rights of women are recognized, this will be symbolically compared with a theocratic patriarchy, where marriage is considered sacred and women are subservient.

Erving Goffman

The symbolic interactionist Erving Goffman (1959) developed what he called the 'dramaturgy'. Human interaction is viewed by Goffman as a dramatic 'performance' (in the acting sense of the term). He argued that society produced 'scripts', guidelines for how to act in the multitudinous roles taken by all members of society. These scripts were internalized through everyday experience, and shaped by the social and physical environment as well as by the reactions of the audience. The environment and the audience provide blatant parameters for what Goffman calls the 'front-stage' performance (for example, written codes of behaviour; consistent positive or negative feedback), while also transmitting rules for the performance obliquely. The front-stage scene is what is presented in public. However, there are also elements to the role being played that are hidden from public view in the 'back-stage'. These elements are the rehearsals, secrets, and deviances of the role.

Front-stage Heather, never wholly consistent in any of her performances, can be fruitfully assertive and amusingly cajoling or, if her script is under-rehearsed, mildly threatening and faintly irritating. However, these mannerisms also surface back-stage. But, like a child without a script who is demanding attention from a parent, or a ham actor desperate for the acclaim of the audience, Heather can over-work her script and become ferocious and exasperating.

With the emergence of globalized mass electronic communication, the drama has entered a virtual world. For example, electronic mail, on-line chat rooms, and specialist internet services (such as those delivering medical advice, or offering therapy sessions) all without face-to-face interaction, carry novel forms of symbolic feedback. Added to this is the increasingly invasive advertising of products that has become an accepted way of generating finance from otherwise unprofitable web-site provision.[3] That is, internet 'pop-ups' are made to be highly symbolic visually to catch the conscious or unconscious attention of the viewer. In electronic communication, the boundaries between front-stage and back-stage areas of a performance become blurred.

The therapy session is a drama. Consider the front-stage: a therapy 'room' conveying selective information to the client: its décor, the chairs or sofas, serene tone, certificates or paintings on the wall, and the box of handkerchiefs. The prestige and power of the therapist are conveyed through the symbols of therapeutic professionalism: the manner in which the client is greeted, a handshake, a smile, a gesture to sit, and now that the scene is set, a cue (verbal or non-verbal) to begin the core theme in this dramatic script – the client's story. Back-stage, however, are the preparations of the therapist and the client prior to the encounter with the client and his/her post-session reflections. Added to this may be deliberate withholding of certain parts of the story being told by the client, kept back-stage because they are too emotionally sensitive or embarrassing. The goal of many therapies, of course, is to enable aspects of the back-stage to enter the front-stage.

Goffman also described how some people undergo 'spoiled identities' because of the stigma from either physical, psychological, or social labels they attract. Regular negative feedback can make an individual feel they are in some way not quite 'normal' or 'whole', because he/she is 'damaged' or 'contaminated'. Self-worth then becomes undermined. A diagnosis of mental disorder or epilepsy, being sent to prison, stuttering, facial disfigurement, or a disability, all may attract stigma and therefore furnish a spoiled identity. In some cultures, an individual may invite a spoiled identity if he/she admits to having had therapy. Heather's impaired self-worth might be attributable to what she read as persistent messages from her father that she wasn't loved as much, or in the same way, as her brother, and that he really wanted another son not a daughter.

Max Weber

Max Weber (1864–1920) was, however, the major instigator of the interactionist perspective in sociology. The underlying philosophies of many other sociological theories also have their origins in his work (especially constructionism and postmodernism). For Weber (1948), humans are experiencing, subjective entities that have consciousness. Metals, planets, protons, cars, neutrons, grass, and air do not think, reflect, and emote. This makes the study of human society a very different feat to that of studying nature and human-made objects.[4] A human being has choices, argues Weber, and constantly elects to make choices. But also for Weber, humans are not unitary organisms operating in a social vacuum. Unlike the reductionism of the psychologist and therapist (and biologist) who addresses human behaviour through the narrow perspective of mental functioning and physiology, Weber perceived humans as inexorably connected to the social setting in which they live out their daily lives, and to the broader society to which they belong. This approach is what he called 'social actionism'.

Weber's social action theory states that the meaning individuals give to their action is what creates society. Society is not, as Durkheim would have it, 'greater than the sum of its parts', but is only 'the sum of its parts'. That is, people react to their environment, and offer interpretations of social events. Therefore, people consciously make and alter the social order around them, rather than, as the structuralists propose, having society impinging on human free will.

Weber rejected 'objective' sociological methods of research. He argued for an 'interpretative' method through which the sociologist would intuitively or empathetically come to understand human behaviour and therefore the working of society. The German word *Verstehen* is commonly used to describe this thorough comprehension of the meaning social actors give to their behaviour. Participant observation is the Weberian research method of choice (although in-depth interviewing is frequently used as a more practical alternative). Here the researcher deliberately enters the world of the people he/she wishes to study. Weber argued that it is only possible to appreciate fully (or as fully as possible) what is happening in any given social situation if you become part of it. At both the individual level, at the larger group level, and structural level, individual and collective interpretations of situations must be understood – then the sociologist has achieved *Verstehen*.

The empathy Weber is referring to is not what therapists mean by the term.[5] Weber's empathy is the tool of the sociological investigator looking for understanding and systematically collating the interpretations of the meanings people give to their performances, as well as what structurally advances or hinders how people perform. The therapist uses empathy as a communication tool; it is operated principally to convey to the client that he/she has a responsive listener.

Weber's academic mission was to challenge the structuralism of Marx. He contradicted Marx by pointing to elements of the superstructure of society (specifically religious belief) operating as the catalyst for change rather than the economic base. Against Marx's historical economic determinism (that is, history changes on the basis of whatever economic system is forming), Weber argued, that it was the sixteenth-century Protestant Reformation in Europe that stimulated the growth of the capitalist mode of production. Specifically, it was the beliefs of the Protestant Calvinists that brought about capitalism.

Calvinists valued hard work and individual achievement. They thought that if their work endeavours were successful and as individuals they advanced in society, then this indicated that God had selected them to enter heaven on death. Crucially, the wealth they accrued could not be spent on 'conspicuous consumption' (which would be sinful), but had to be reinvested in business and commerce. This had the effect, reasoned Weber, of building up the industrial economies of Europe, which then stimulated capitalist growth in other parts of the world.

Weber also disagreed with Marx over who had power in society. Marx pinpointed the locus of power is society as in the hands of the dominant economic group (that is, a ruling class who owned the means of production whether this be during antiquity, feudalism, or capitalism). But Weber believed that people other than those with economic supremacy could hold power in society. Weber's point was that certain 'status groups' may have more esteem and influence than the wealthy owners of business and commerce. For example, in liberal democracies, an individual born at the bottom of the social hierarchy can (in theory) rise to the top by gaining educational and professional qualifications. The daughter of a road-sweeper could become a doctor or lawyer, or the son of a factory worker could be a Prime Minister or President. Winning the lottery might not mean automatic entry into the power elite of a society, but will alter the social prestige of the winner or his/her offspring. In totalitarian societies, subterfuge may be used by revolutionary groups to remove those in power and allow a new group to dominate. Gramsci (1971), who was imprisoned in the late 1920s and early 1930s by the Italian fascist leader Mussolini, wrote about how to replace fascism with socialism. A 'war of manoeuvre' (a frontal attack on an enemy) *or* a 'war of position' (political and cultural movements, and the education of the masses), could bring about the new regime. That is, Gramsci, although a Marxist, did recognize that social change could occur through the relatively measured campaigns of interest groups (in this case, it was the Communists) rather than only through abrupt, intense and more than likely violent upheaval.

Groups of people can employ a 'war of position', not to change the ruling regime, but to increase their control over their own work and gain greater remuneration and employment perks. The medical and legal professions have done this successfully. Physiotherapy, occupational therapy, audiology, clinical psychology, and nursing have attempted to repeat the success of medicine and law. Therapy has joined in the game of social repositioning. The technique used by such groups, argued Weber, is that of 'social closure'. In order to advance the status of a group, its leaders make it increasingly difficult to belong to that group by elevating the requirements for entry. Furthermore, the claim is advanced by the group that only *its* members have the authority and expertise to operate in a well-defined area of work (such as surgery and prescribing, and legal representation and judgement).

Weber's sociology has made notable contributions to social policy. For example, many government health programmes in Britain have included a modification to the crude idea that simply telling people what to do about their health (for example, stop smoking, stop drinking, and stop being a couch potato) will work equally for all social groups. It has become *de rigueur* to try to understand why certain social groups persist in unhealthy behaviour in order then to make health promotion tactics more effective.

Furthermore, Weber's notion of social status has been used by policy-makers in Britain to categorize the population into occupational groups. Throughout the twentieth century, the Registrar General placed occupations within a social status hierarchy, which enabled researchers and governments to assess structural trends in, for example, employment, crime, residence, and health. The use of a standard measure of occupational status also allows statistics to be compared historically and geographically. The Registrar General's schema contained five categories, ranging from professional to unskilled occupations. However, by the end of the twentieth century these categories and their order were becoming invalid because certain occupations had improved or worsened their social status, and a swathe of new occupations had come about. Consequently, another system for allocating occupations was invented, but this still follows Weber's conceptualization of social status. Since 2001, the National Statistics Socio-economic Classification (NS-SEC) has been used for official statistics and surveys (Office for National Statistics 2005).

Classification systems used by governments and researchers are relevant to therapy. For example, they provide information on psychiatric epidemiology and mental health inequalities in incidence and take-up of services including therapy (Pilgrim and Rogers 2002).

Constructionism

The interactionist places the individual at the centre of sociological analysis, but still recognizes how individuals and social structures affect each other. However, the notion that individuals give 'meaning' to their lives is taken much further by constructionist theorists. For the constructionist, the social world does not have an unadulterated objective existence. All social phenomena are to a greater or lesser extent 'constructed'. Things become 'real' only through humans attaching particular meanings to them. To use Peter Berger and Thomas Luckmann's (1966) seminal phrase, 'reality is socially constructed'.

In this point of view, diseases and states of mind are human fabrications. They do not exist without someone recognizing and defining them. Whereas the medical scientist believes that diseases actually exist and can be identified and described as 'facts', the constructionist argues that they only have the appearance of having a reality because of the coming together of certain historical and social processes. At other times, and in other places, they would either not be construed as real at all or they would be interpreted as different entities.

There is a link between 'cultural relativism' and constructionism. If social phenomena are manufactured by socially produced values, then the worth of cultural practices other than our own cannot be judged on the basis of 'right' and 'wrong', or 'better' and 'worse'. Each culture can only be assessed in its own terms. We cannot declare that a set of beliefs and behaviours from another culture, no matter how virtuous or abhorrent they seem to us, merits either replicating in our culture or needs to be eradicated in that culture. Consequently, whether it's the ritualistic expunging of the clitoris in young North African women, the pervasive death penalty in China, or human rights abuses in Middle Eastern countries, there can be no justification for moral outrage, or universal laws on human conduct.

Labelling

Constructionism has been a major influence in theorizing about social deviancies, including mental disorder and psychological distress generally, in the form of 'labelling theory' (or 'social reaction' theory). Labelling theory examines what is categorized as 'deviance' in society (for example, criminality, madness, and what has been tagged by many Western governments as 'anti-social behaviour'). It considers deviance not in terms of the inherent biological or psychological characteristics of the individual malefactor, but as sets of actions or beliefs which attract the tag of 'deviancy' (Lemert 1951; Becker 1963). What the labelling theorists argue is that an action is not in itself either 'normal' or 'abnormal' until that meaning has been ascribed to it by the powerful groups in society. Being a 'good citizen' is dependent upon the creation of a social contract by politicians that prescribes what a 'good citizen' means. Different political parties will have different views. Car theft, burglary, or even murder, are not crimes until the criminal justice system declares them to be so. Eating too much, drinking too much, smoking, and being indolent are not abhorrent behaviours until the 'health police' decide they are.

Many crimes are never categorized as crimes because they have not been observed by those with the power to denote that label. People who carry out criminal actions do not become criminals if they are not caught, prosecuted, and found guilty. Moreover, law-breaking (speeding, running red lights, under-age drinking, under-age sex, and using illegal 'recreational' drugs) constantly occurs and is done by a high percentage of the population, but unless there is a social reaction to the individual rule-breaker (for example, he/she is arrested by the police), then a criminal label is not assigned.

Labels matter because they affect social attitudes and self-identity. However, a distinction can be made between primary and secondary stages of labelling. Rule-breaking has only a negligible effect on how rule-breakers perceive themselves or are viewed by others. This is especially the case if our deviancy is unnoticed by the powerful. But if our actions are discovered and the reaction of others is marked, we might begin a 'deviant career' (Goffman 1963). The secondary stage of labelling is entered whereby, because of consistent reinforcement of the label, a permanent deviant identity is forged. The label then starts to define the person, and he/she internalizes the performance that is connected to that label. Furthermore, the process of becoming a complete deviant is enhanced if the individual socializes with groups who have been given similar labels. 'Total institutions', such as gaol and asylums will reinforce a criminal or mad identity (Goffman 1961).

Postmodernism

The constructionist argument is that although social phenomena are not 'real', this does not mean that they are not experienced as real. Humans construct their realities by objectifying subjective experience (Berger and Luckman 1966). Social phenomena are imbued with culturally pertinent value and utility. They therefore have a (constructed) vital capacity which is both produced by society and is necessary for society to operate. We live our lives as though war, money, friendship, fatherhood, holidays, the law, and health have a tangible existence even if they can be deconstructed and reformulated by academics and shown not to be what they were originally perceived to be.

However, postmodernist ideas (again not a united perspective) take constructionism further. For the postmodernist, everything in not only the social word but also the physical world, the universe(s), and whatever else might be beyond and behind what we presently understand as factual is an 'interpretation' of the human mind. There are no, and can never be, any universal laws or incontrovertible established facts. Truth of any sort, therefore, is not possible, ever.

The legitimacy of the 'grand narratives' (for example, nationhood, Christianity, Islam, Judaism, socialism, capitalism, and science) that purported to explain the social, physical or spiritual world, has been supplanted. There has also been a reduction in the degree of deference shown formerly to leaders, experts, teachers, the police and the judiciary, and the clergy.

What we know about black holes, DNA, genes, molecules, fruit flies, the sun, Pluto, hamsters, Australians, beauty, hate, hypertension, and cancer, is only 'known' in the way it is because we perceive it as such. Nothing whatsoever, therefore, exists (or at least has the existence we believe it to have) independent of the human mind. The natural or social world is described using meanings and symbols that have their origins in particular social processes. Without the European Enlightenment, there would not be the vocabulary or technologies that have shaped the Western outlook on physical and chemical matter, the connection between causes and effects, and how the body and mind become diseased. Consequently, 'science' itself cannot be separated from the social processes (which encompass not only the Enlightenment but a range of social factors from Graeco-Roman beliefs to the way in which politicians orchestrate what it is they wish to have researched).

Such a view of the social and physical world implies that there are no inherently good or bad ways of living our lives, and we live in a 'cultural marketplace' that reconstructs humans as 'consumers' to choose a way of living from an endless array of possibilities (Crook et al. 1992). Moreover, all aspects of social life (for example, health, holidays, sex, entertainment, leisure, and death) have become 'commodities'.

Visits to the health food shop to sniff or bathe in aromatic oils or to waft herbs at our torments are as common as attendance at the general practitioner's surgery for a bottle of pink medicine or box of white pills. Science and astrology are consulted for their prophetic explication on an equal footing. Existential reprogramming, holotropic breathwork, bionomic harmonizing, and Rolfing, sit alongside cognitive-behaviourism in the postmodern psycho-market.

Heather's lifestyle could be described as postmodern. She mixes the arguably culturally elevated activities of concert attendance, high educational attainment, and a refusal to own a television with the perhaps less edifying cultural habits of shooting pool, having little grasp on world events, and binge drinking. Moreover, Heather's divergent emotional, cognitive, and behavioural traits are a representation of the 'postmodern personality'.

Such choice over who we want to be, and what we want to do, can be empowering or disabling. It can either bring a sense of absolute freedom, or induce what the existentialist philosopher (who was also, paradoxically, a Marxist) Jean-Paul Sartre described as '*La Nausée*' (translated as 'The Nausea').[6]

La Nausée is a psycho-social condition whereby humans come to realize (helped to such a startling insight perhaps by existential therapy) that human existence is absurd and meaningless. Sartre's diary-writing fictional character in *La Nausée*, Monsieur Antoine Roquentin, describes his existential awaking thus:

> Something has happened to me: I can't doubt it any more. It came as an illness does, not like an ordinary certainty, not like anything obvious. It installed itself cunningly, little by little; I felt a little strange, a little awkward, and that was all. Once it was established, it didn't move any more, it lay low and I was able to persuade myself that there was nothing wrong with me, that is was false alarm. And now it has started blossoming.
>
> (Sartre [1938] 1965: 13)

Monsieur Roquentin, as *La Nausée* invades his consciousness, muses 'I am beginning to believe that nothing can ever be proved' (1965: 26). He then comes to grasp the social basis to his psychological condition and exclaims, 'The Nausea isn't inside me ... it is I who am inside *it*' (1965: 26).

Similarly, Heather's existential angst (the insecurity and fear of rejection), seemingly so deeply ingrained in her own psyche, may actually stem from the uncertainties and choices in postmodern society.

Michel Foucault provided the basis for the nihilistic tendency of postmodernist thinking. This is obvious when his controversial (to say the least) claim that 'man did not exist' before the eighteenth century is examined. According to Foucault (1966), 'the human' as an individual was an invention of the nineteenth century, brought about by concepts, language, and technologies (what Foucault described as 'discourses') from the emerging disciplines of biology, psychology, linguistics, *and* sociology. It was the discourses of these disciplines that re-constructed humans from being identified with nature and as interlinked segments of groups (for example, families and cultures) to unitary and unique beings.

Some therapists have used the social constructionist perspective (for example, McNamee and Gergen 1992; Hedges 2005). The view is taken by social constructionist therapists that humans can come to understand and then alter their socially given 'narratives' (that is, the stories they tell to make sense of their lives) about who they are and what they can achieve. Such therapists attempt to rise above the utter nihilism of the postmodern position, but do agree that ambiguity abounds. Their message to clients is that ambiguity in life should be accepted but managed if necessary. We live in a messy world[7] (in such spheres as morality and politics), and learning to live with chaos may be an essential strategy in order to find psychological stability.

Realism

Realism attempts a synthesis of the otherwise antagonistic perspectives of, on the one hand, structuralism/science, and, on the other, interactionism/constructionism. For the realist, there are 'real' things in the natural and social world that can eventually be known, but it is damned difficult to find them. This is because of how human culture spawns beliefs that confuse what is real and what is false. Added to this problem of the cultural overlay on 'facts' is the inadequacy of social and natural scientific technique to date. The task of establishing truth in the social and natural world therefore is doubly hindered.

Best guess

So, in the natural world there are concrete objects and universal laws, but humans can only experience these subjectively and therefore can never 'know' in the purest sense anything. Science offers us a 'best guess' of what these objects are and how the world operates. The realist also posits that humans are both shaped by, and help shape, their social world. That is, humans have a reflexive relationship with society. What an individual feels, does and thinks affects the content and form of social processes, and the way in which society is structured. Equally, social processes and structures configure the circumstances under which human performance is expressed. Consequently, neither the human performance nor society remains static. Changes in both, while not necessarily random and amorphous, are not unilinear and are therefore difficult to predict, as is identifying in the first place why people feel, act, and think in particular ways and society operates as it does. But in the future, sociology, psychology (and therapy) might be able to understand fully, or prophesy accurately, human performance and social phenomena.

The continuous re-arranging and updating of social and scientific knowledge (and periodic paradigm shifts) are indicative of the relatively primitive methods available for discovering reality, as is the common occurrence of contrary research findings. One study suggests drinking alcohol is beneficial to health, while another either alters the recommended amount or concludes that alcohol should not be taken medicinally at all as it does more harm than good; one study implies that teaching children to read and write at an early age is essential for later educational attainment and therefore employment opportunities, but another argues for play to be encouraged as social intelligence will be far more useful in succeeding in life. With regard to therapy, cognitive-behaviourism has much supportive evidence and became the vogue therapy in the 2000s, but it may in future years be found to have only a narrow and short-term effect and consequently lose favour.

Transitive and instransitive knowledge

The realist Roy Bhaskar (1998) offers a way of comprehending this discrepancy between what we think we know about the social and natural worlds and what actually is in these worlds. For Bhaskar, there are two forms of knowledge. First, there is what he describes as 'intransitive knowledge'. Intransitive knowledge is made up of the invariable facts that exist with or without our knowledge of them. Second, there is transitive knowledge. Transitive knowledge is made up of the language, concepts, and technologies of the epistemological discourse that is afforded credibility in a specific culture or epoch to tackle reality. Today, it is science that dominates as an explanatory paradigm (although a conglomeration of major and minor religions still attempt to explain the meaning of the social and natural worlds, and the postmodernists regard explanation as an epistemological free-for-all).

But does truth matter? Ophelia Benson and Jeremy Stangroom (2006) argue vehemently that it does. They attack what they describe as the 'assorted political and ideological agendas' in academia, especially postmodernism) that they suggest have made truth unfashionable. Cynicism about truth has been fuelled by the premeditated misinterpretation of science:

It is arguable that obfuscation is what postmodernism is all about. Clouds of squid ink in the form of jargon, mathematical equations whose relevance is obscure, peacock displays of name-dropping, misappropriation and misapplication of scientific theories are often seen in postmodernist 'discourse'. Nietzsche, Heidegger, Heisenberg, Einstein, Godel, Wittgenstein are hauled in and cited as saying things they didn't say.

(Benson and Stangroom 2006: 9)

Benson and Stangroom are highly critical of a general intellectual laziness which leads to truth being ignored or not sought, and of the bastardization of truth by religious fundamentalists.

The overall message from Benson and Stangroom is that not all opinions concerning the social and natural world are equal, and that science has a long pedigree of truth-seeking. Facts exist, and cannot be open to other interpretations. They cite the murder of millions throughout history in the many instances of massacres, war crimes and ethnic cleansings.

However, from a realist perspective, murder *is* open to other interpretations. For example, humans killing humans can be categorized as criminal or legal, or morally justified or unwarranted, depending on how it is perceived. There is the reality of a dead body (or bodies) but the event of killing can be considered in alternative ways (Morrall 2006a).

Summary

The sociological imagination invites a broader appreciation of human problems than has traditionally been forthcoming from therapy. Humans and their social environment cannot be separated. Human problems, for the sociologist, are either born of society or have a strong connection to society.

Stucturalist sociology challenges therapists to do much more than navel-gaze with the client. For the structuralist, there is a patent need to see the individual as a part of a social system, and increasingly as belonging to a global village. Ultimately, the structuralist takes the view that society has to be altered, perhaps radically, before many human problems can be resolved.

The interactionist sociologist also pays homage to the power humans have as individuals, to make their own meanings about their lives rather than having these meanings thrust upon from society. It is they who make up society, and have the power to influence society (more plausibly when they act rather than being passive. But there is still a society in which interaction takes place, and which sets the scene for the type of script which individuals can improvise.

Constructionist sociology, and its extremist offspring postmodernism, attempt to debunk reality by suggesting that there is an infinitive number of realities. Humans therefore can either celebrate their liberty to manufacture a personalized lifestyle, self-identity, and belief system, or degenerate into a condition of downright nothingness, hopelessness, and cynicism.

Finally, the realist sociologist wants to mend epistemological fences. For the realist, there really is a reality, a truth, and facts. Developments in neurobiology are leading to interesting philosophical debates about free will and the unconscious cerebral mechanisms which may determine decision-making (Frith 2007; Hind 2007).

However, we await the methods (scientific or otherwise) that will eventually expunge completely the cultural attributes that are attached to reality, truths, facts, and free will. When (and if) this happens, the real, truthful and factual nature of human problems is exposed, then therapy can be appropriately re-designed.

Enlightenment about how society affects human performance (including the troubles of Heather) is obtained from whichever sociological perspective is embraced. For example, an individual's feelings of insecurity and rejection cannot be divorced from the social (and physical) environment in which he/she exists. But, how potent the effect of society is considered to be on an individual, and the perceived ability of that individual to manage him/herself in society, will depend on which perspective is selected. Given the perspectives presented above, Heather can be comprehended as a product of society, a producer of society, or product *and* a producer.

CHAPTER 2

Dysfunctional

Conflict
Lottery
Rivalry

If therapy was a family or an individual and came to the attention of social services it is probable that it would be classified as dysfunctional and put on an 'at risk' register.

Going against the standard proposition from sociological functionalism that considers all social institutions as advantageous to society, functionalist Robert Merton (1957) recognizes that some social institutions harm society. For Merton, these institutions are injurious because they are riddled with 'struggles'. The therapeutic enterprise is so riddled.

On the surface, therapy seems to contain little controversy. There are clear expositions of its theories and practices of therapy available from a vast number of sources.[1] Moreover, therapy agencies and theorists project a transparent *raison d'être*. Therapy, it is suggested by its advocates, is aimed manifestly at providing help for individuals, couples, or groups who want to resolve personal problems which are causing psychological distress. Therapists, such an undemanding portrayal continues, gain their knowledge, skills, and attitudes about being helpful through designated training courses and supervision of their practice. Advanced courses and intense supervision presumably make the therapist outstandingly helpful.

But the trouble with therapy is that if one digs a bit deeper into the dirt of the therapeutic enterprise with the sharp shovel of scepticism, then what is uncovered is not soil enriched with clarity, consent and compassion, but mud befouled by confusion, competitiveness, and confrontation.

By 'therapeutic enterprise' I mean the totality of:

1   practices (what the therapist does with the client);
2   knowledge (the perspectives of therapy furnished mainly by psychology, but with contributions from, for example, social psychology, psychiatry, and neurology);
3   people (the practitioners and their supervisors, and the clients);
4   agencies (the training, and registration/membership organizations);
5   paraphernalia (for example, the American Psychological Association[2] (2008) lists 1,844 topics under the search-term 'psychotherapy': along with types of therapy and the different client groups who may require specialist therapies, audio-visual packages about therapy, therapy training manuals, and therapy journals and books, are listed in their hundreds).

The concept of the therapeutic enterprise indicates that therapy is about much more than simply helping people. It is a complex, commercial, amorphous, escalating, factional, and dissolute social phenomenon. This is rich pickings indeed for the sociologically imaginative and troublesome sceptic, and grist to the mill for Heather's fiery scorn.

Sociological points about specific aspects of the therapeutic enterprise are made in this chapter. But, in the main, sociological observations about the therapeutic enterprise as a whole are offered. I accept that any sweeping commentary about therapy does give weight to the accusations of caricaturing and generalizing. But this, I argue, is legitimate because any critique would have an impossible task if it attempted to appraise all areas of therapy in one book. More crucially, the social phenomenon of therapy, notwithstanding its complexity, commercialism, amorphousness, escalation, factionalism, and dissolution, can be appreciated 'from the outside' as having grand effects in a similar way to observing a storm cloud. The meteorologist will want to know the intricate molecular actions of the nimbostratus. But for most other people, foretelling that torrential rain, bolts of lightning, and thunderous noise are likely to ensue from this dark and nebulous canopy is good enough. Moreover, just as the bursting of the violent deluge has benefits (watering the countryside and sweeping away the detritus of the city) and drawbacks (flooding the land and the occasional death), so therapy may enrich humanity (nourishing the soul) but can also cause damage (debilitating society).

First, the history of therapy is traced, a history that illuminates major *conflicts* in the embryonic development of the therapeutic enterprise, ones that remain apparent. But discord in the therapeutic enterprise is not confined to the residual effects from its early days. Alongside, remaining definitional disputes (about what therapy is, who should be a therapist, and the differences between psychotherapy and counselling), there are new and growing tensions over the *lottery* involved in selecting a therapy and therapist, as well as a good deal of *rivalry* among the plethora of therapy agencies.

Conflict

The histories of psychotherapy and counselling reveal the good intentions of those endeavouring to tackle human psychological distress, and no sceptical review of therapy, sociological or otherwise, should ignore or downgrade the genuineness of these attempts (certainly not, I suggest, without offering alternatives). However, unpicking the historical background of therapy also sheds light on a dark side not only of humanity but also of therapy, revealing the struggles for domination, professional empire-building, pomposity and self-delusion, the settling of personal scores, and what seem with hindsight very dubious practices.

Throughout the hundreds of thousands of years of human history, people have used verbal and non-verbal communication to pay attention to each other's psyche. After all, that is what language is all about, the giving and receiving of messages indicating what is on your or the other person's mind. Moreover, language has always been used to resolve human problems, for example, as a warning of danger, in the search for food, and obtaining a mate. It is well established that in ancient societies (Egyptian, Greek, and Roman), and from the Enlightenment onwards in the West, the psychological needs of humans have been realized and treated not just with medicines but with talk (Freedheim 1992). There are historical examples of cultures formulating sophisticated therapeutic psychologies. Sufism, the eighth-century mystical offshoot of Islam which is thriving today, means 'healing of the soul'. The Sufi Psychology Association (2007) advocates and dispenses through conferences, literature, and retreats, a spiritual brand of psychotherapy for soul healing.

Freud's dangerous ideas

It was, however, Sigmund Freud (1856–1939), who in the late Victorian era gave the intellectual and procedural base necessary for modern psychotherapy. This was the time when European and North American scientific, technological, medical, and social innovation abounded. Originality in psychology, therefore, was to be expected. Freud most certainly delivered a package of considerations about the human psyche that contained such novel elements that it stretched the public's imagination to the same extent as Charles Darwin (1809–1882) has done with his premise of natural selection in the origin of the species (1859).

Just as Darwin had shocked Victorian society by linking apes to humans through his account of evolution, so did Freud's dissection of human sexuality. He covered: infantile sexuality; violence and sexuality; death and sexuality; female sexuality; masturbation; anal eroticism; bisexuality; incest and the Oedipal Complex; homosexuality; defloration as social 'branding'; the totemic and taboo social value of virginity; sexual sadism and masochism (Young-Bruehl 2006; Gay 2006).

As Richard Dawkins and Stephen Pinker observe (in Brockman 2007), human civilization (which for them is one supported by scientific evidence and rational argument) progresses through 'dangerous ideas' that offend 'collective decency' and undercut the 'safe' ideas of a particular era. Destabilizing the moral order of accepted knowledge is likely to incur the wrath and ridicule of the guardians of morality and knowledge. But like Darwin, Freud was not easily dismissed as a crank. Both were meticulous and methodical in their work, both had considerable intellects, and carried with them the aura of scientific respectability and ingenuity because they *were* scientists, Darwin the botanist and Freud the neurologist.

Freud practised medicine from 1886 to 1896. However, he had become increasingly intrigued by one side of his practice, neurotic illness. Previously, Freud had worked under the eminent neurologist Jean-Martin Charcot at the Salpêtrière Hospital in Paris. Charcot's interest was in hysteria ('conversion disorder'), which he regarded as a disorder of the mind but one which was caused by hereditary disorder. Charcot's mentorship of Freud was to stimulate the latter's fascination with hysteria.

Hysteria had already attracted some peculiar diagnoses and treatments. Hippocrates assumed hysteria was caused by the womb escaping its moorings in the pelvis and wandering around the unfortunate woman's body. Apart from hypnosis, which was favoured by Charcot, medical practitioners might digitally manipulate the genitals, apply a vibrator, or conduct 'water massage', for the purpose of inducing an orgasm which was thought to be effective in relieving hysteria (Maines 1999).

Freud's work reinforced sex as central to hysteria and other neuroses. But he was determined to discover a more sophisticated reason for the fainting attacks, bouts of blindness and paralysis, bizarre postures, facial contortions, and vaginal spasms of his young female patients when there was no apparent organic causation other than a lack of sexual climax. What Freud experimented with was 'talk': prompting patients to tell their life stories and picking up on clues of psychological pathology via their dreams, slips of the tongue, evasiveness, and defensiveness. He called his talking therapy 'psychoanalysis'.

Freud wanted a new *science* of the mind. But, despite his medical background, his scientific conviction that true knowledge came about from establishing cause and effect relationships, the rigour in his investigations, and his view (similar to that of Karl Marx's) that religion was an illusion, it takes a gigantic leap of faith to accept psychoanalysis as a 'science'. Anthony Storr, psychiatrist, therapist, and academic, is not persuaded:

He [Freud] called the system which he invented [psychoanalysis] a science; but is not, could never have been, a science in the sense in which physics or chemistry are sciences, since its hypotheses are retrospective and cannot be used for prediction, and most are insusceptible to final proof.

(Storr 2001)

This lack of scientific credibility haunts psychoanalysis, especially in Western and Westernized health care systems where empirical ('evidence-based') justification has become mandatory in the formulation of policy *about*, but not always *in*, practice. Moreover, psychoanalysis, digging as it does deep into childhood experiences and unconscious mechanisms, is too long term for health care services fixated on cost-effectiveness.

Rather than viewed as a science, psychoanalysis can be seen as a doctrinal forerunner of the array of New Age religions and alternative medicines that flourished at the end of the twentieth century and into the twenty-first century in the West. Psychoanalysis may, therefore, be just another cult or 'snake oil' like Neo-paganism and homeopathy, depending for its declared legitimacy on nothing more than assertion and the zeal of its exponents. Richard Webster (2005) considers psychoanalysis to be a secular substitute for religion, a messianic creed dressed up as science.

But psychotherapy cannot be so easily dismissed as, say, anthropomancy, alchemy, astrology, or aromatherapy. Freudian ideas are persistent, pervasive, and prominent. That is, they have become culturally embedded. Moreover, Freud's treatment (at least for hysteria) appeared to work.

Freud's feuds

Freud was to carry out lecture tours on psychoanalysis in Europe and North America, and write prolifically about his patients. In doing so he gained a multitude of disciples and collaborators who spread his theories across the Western and civilized world. Unfortunately, not only did he upset the medical and psychiatric establishment, he was eventually to fall out with most of his former allies. But before he did, Freud managed to set up a number of psychoanalytic institutions, which have survived into the twenty-first century.

Freud and his acolytes would meet regularly during 1902 on a Wednesday, so, with ineffable logic they decided to call these gatherings 'The Psychological Wednesday Society'. By 1908, the name had become 'The Vienna Psychoanalytical Society', presumably because they usually met in Vienna and on days other than Wednesday. The 'First Congress for Freudian Psychology' was also held that year in Salzburg, and two years later the second Congress was held in Nuremberg. Freud wanted to spread his ideas to other countries, and under his influence the International Psychoanalytical Association was founded.

However, there are numerous contending psychoanalytical organizations, which were either formed by erstwhile devotees of Freud (such as Joseph Breuer, Wilhelm Stekel, Wilhelm Fliess, Carl Jung, and Alfred Adler) or by 'post-Freudian' therapists (specifically, the psychodynamic therapists, all of whom owe their theoretical roots to Freud, but disagree with one or more aspects of his original formulations). The disagreements were often vitriolic (Grosskurth 1991). This was in part due to Freud's obsessive commitment to his own formulations, and his tendency to rile even his close collaborators by ignoring or over-ruling their moderating or alternative opinions.

In particular, Freud and Jung's close partnership in the promotion and dissemination of psychoanalysis disintegrated into absurd animosity. Accusations abounded, and hostile letters were sent between the two over many years. Much of the antagonism was oriented around the subject of sex. Jung remonstrated that Freud over-emphasized sexuality as a prime motivator in human behaviour, and each accused the other of sexual indiscretions. Some of these accusations are credible. It was well known at the time that Jung had adulterous affairs with a colleague and patients

(Carotenuto 1984). Then, in 2007, Franz Maciejewski, while researching a book on Freud, found a guest book at a Swiss hotel which implicated Freud in a sexual relationship with his sister-in-law (Follain 2007).

But Freud and Jung also didn't agree about the nature of incest, dreams, religion, and occultism. Moreover, their personal relationship contained a 'father-and-son' imbalance (which the 'son' Jung came to resent) and love–hate ambivalence (the feeling of both men changing regularly, but eventually resting on mutual detestation). As though that was not enough, Oedipus stalked their relationship (Jung's latter-day criticisms of Freud's ideas seen by the latter as an attempt by the 'son' to slay the 'father'), as unresolved homosexuality (with Jung's original admiration of Freud having undertones of sexual desire) (McGuire 1974; Donn 1988).

It is not the Oedipal complex but its father-daughter equivalent, the Electra complex that Heather's Jungian-orientated therapist wanted to explore. The libidinous attachment of a daughter to her father as a psychological stage during childhood was proposed first by Freud but named and given more importance by Jung (1966). As soon as Heather became aware that this was the direction this therapist wished to head, she abandoned him (after only two sessions).

Len, Heather's barefoot therapist, who had recommended the Jungian, was disappointed but not surprised that any investigation of the relationship she had with her father would not be welcome. He had believed for a long time that the ultimate resolution to Heather's troubles would have to do just this, but that she would resist such scrutiny. He, from his cursory reading of Freud and Jung, understood that when daughters becomes stuck at this stage, they may as an adult seek out male sexual mates who have similar personalities and physiques to their fathers. Or they may go in the opposite direction and seek men who are completely unlike the fathers they could not possess and be possessed by (and Heather took this route with relationships during her teens). Len, some 15 years older than Heather, may well have represented the father-figure she longed for (an idealization of her real father). Saint, her first husband, was not authoritarian like her father, but had many qualities similar to those of her father, especially his constrained emotional expressiveness. But, not showing enough affection, Heather had told Len, was a major reason for her to abandon that marriage. Just what will happen in her marriage to Damian, husband number two (five years Heather's senior but with a much older performance), depends on the pliability of his personality. If he is unable to tread the fine line between being too much like Heather's real father and too little like his idealized version, he may also be abandoned.

Freud's legacy

After the death, Freud was (and is) neither forgotten nor forgiven. Freud managed to attract immense fury, and some of the most ferocious attacks came from sociologists. It is not hard to understand why. Hordes of fuming feminists have long held him culpable of giving credence to extreme sexism and patriarchy. Certainly, Freud's work can be read as regarding women as failed, underdeveloped, and irrational versions of men. Undeniably, he did propose that women were obsessively envious of men's penises, the libido was basically a masculine drive that women somehow borrowed from men, and women, because of their core biological make-up, were for ever in danger of succumbing to mental derangement (Young-Bruel 1990).

However, other sociologists have seen much merit in Freud's work for the connection that is made between the individual and society. Robert Bocock (1977) argues that Freud *was* a sociologist. For Bocock, Freud appreciates the influence of society on the development of the personality, and in particular the socialization of the super-ego (that is, the individual's 'conscience'). Freud's view of human sexuality, that it was 'polymorphously perverse', was an indictment of biological determinism (and, by implication, of contemporary neo-evolutionary theory). The many facets of sexual desire and enactment Freud recorded affirmed that sexuality in humans expanded way beyond heterosexual genital conjoining necessary for procreation. Baby-making was only part of what humans wanted from sex. However, a society, either through a repressive or liberal moral code, shapes how sexuality is manifested. Specifically, the raw biological instinct of sexuality (Eros), as well as that of destruction (Thanatos), *has* to be culturally managed. Freud's work can contribute sociologically as well as psychologically to an analysis of the new sexualities and refashioning of sexualities in the twenty-first century global village.

Although, according to Jerry Adler (2006), Freud is the most 'debunked doctor' in modern times, he is still embedded in Western society. From Freud, argues Alder, Western society has not only inherited 'talking' as a recognized way of dealing with psychological distress and an acceptance of the existence and power of the unconscious, but an array of concepts popular with therapists and/or the wider populace. These include: slips of the tongue; defence mechanisms; the Oedipus complex; and free association.

Uppity counselling

Further fraught infighting among the therapy fraternity was to dissect the therapeutic enterprise. Although Freud's support for therapists who were not medically trained was incontestable, the increasing might of the medical profession in the USA in the early part of the twentieth century influenced who could and who could not be legally described as a psychoanalyst (and by default, a psychotherapist). Using a tactic that has served the medical and other professions well, an area of work (in this case, the professional treatment of psychological distress) was closed off to anyone other than those whom the professionals decided was suitably qualified. For example, in the 1920s, the American Medical Association took a position of non-cooperation with those who were not psychiatrists, and New York State outlawed lay (that is, non-medical) therapy altogether (IPA 2007).

But sometimes, such strategies (what Max Weber described as 'social closure': Weber 1948) backfire spectacularly. It was Carl Rogers (1902–87) who was to spawn a separate non-medical wing of therapy. He was a non-medically trained therapist who in order to keep practising re-branded what he did as 'counselling'. From that point onwards, medical control over therapy was lost.

Ernesto Spinelli (1994) records that counselling is a term that had been used to indicate purposeful interpersonal interactions, and different con-notations of the term remain, ranging from helping to admonishing. But its contemporary therapeutic meaning was formulated by Rogers. Rogers' approach challenged further the medical underpinnings of therapy. Rather than a 'doctor knows best' relationship with the 'patient', Rogers put for-ward a schema that not only suggested non-psychiatrists could become therapists, but that 'patients' should be viewed as 'clients' who had as much if not more to contribute to the conditions under which therapy operated. Rogers was opposed to psychoanalysis (and also behaviourism) because the power was in the hands of the doctor to direct the agenda of the therapy session. His humanistic 'client-centred' (which he was to re-label 'person-centred') therapy was to be 'non-directive'. The client's story (his/her own account of whatever was causing him/her psychological distress), told at a pace decided by the client, was to be the focus of the therapy session. The therapist's contribution was to encourage the telling of the story by unconditionally respecting the client as a person, and by being genuine and honest with the client. Rogers believed that it is only when clients are treated in this way do they have the potential to solve personal problems and have the possibility of reaching a unique nirvana of personal growth (that is, 'self-actualization').

All of this raised the authority of client and lowered that of the therapist, and medical practitioners have been historically greatly opposed to anything that lowers their prestige. However, it was to get worse for the medical profession. They had lost control over the business of psychological distress through the creation of counselling, but eventually anyone could describe themselves as a therapist or, if necessary, take a course to allow him/her to become registered as such with non-medical organizations. Of course, the authority of psychiatry, while not unscathed by this and other threats to its dominance, has been re-affirmed to a large extent through physical therapies (psychotropic medication, psychosurgery, and electro-convulsive therapy) *and* through a continued embracing of talking therapies.

But there remains a persistent attitude from the public (as well from within sections of the enterprise of therapy) that counselling, because of its 'de-medicalized' heritage, is inferior to psychotherapy. The American Counseling Association (2007) points out that this prejudice is ironic as Rogers believed in science and conducted empirical research into his patient's psychological states. However, it is very questionable as to whether the (supposed) rigours of scientific medicine were, or could be, reproduced by Rogers. His humanistic suppositions about empathy, trust, congruity, genuineness, honesty, and unconditional positive regard, and self-actualization certainly have moral worth. But they are inherently 'phenomenological' qualities. That is, they are personal attributes which have meaning for the individual but are not susceptible to standardized measurement, generalization, and prediction. That is, they are not easily testable scientifically.

There was also a drift by Rogers during his career away from science towards constructionism, if not mysticism (O'Hara 1995). Furthermore, Rogers' suppositions are culturally bound, emanating as they did from a particularly liberalizing epoch in the USA, and hence do not necessarily resonate with the moral codes of other societies and perhaps not even in the USA in the twenty-first century.

Spinelli (1994) observes that practitioners who describe themselves as psychotherapists rather than counsellors (and who may have chosen to undertake a 'psychotherapy' training course rather than one in 'counselling'), may be doing so in the assumption that this provides a higher status. But for him there *is* no actual difference between the two, and he accepts the interchangeable uses of the terms. Both have the same goals (roughly translated as the resolution of personal problems, and making steps towards personal change), share theoretical constructs, and give high importance to the 'therapeutic relationship' between therapist and client.

But Spinelli appreciates that, for the public, counselling clearly has populist appeal, while psychotherapy appears, by contrast, elitist. Psychotherapy, perhaps because it has historically been used as a synonym for psychoanalysis, is considered longer-term and more intensive than counselling.

However, Spinelli's own therapeutic identity has all angles covered. He is a Professor of Psychotherapy, Counselling and Counselling Psychology, fellow of the British Counselling Association for Counselling and Psychotherapy (BACP), fellow of the British Psychological Society (BPS), and a United Kingdom Council for Psychotherapy (UKCP) registered psychotherapist.

Definitional indistinctness

Moreover, Spinelli's (all-be-it qualified) belief that today there is little discernible distinction between counselling and psychotherapy is not always what some therapy agencies claim. Real or imagined contrasts have been, and still are, declared by these agencies. For example, Hans Hoxter (1999), the then Honorary Life President of the International Association for Counselling, admits that there is uncertainty about what psychotherapists do that counsellors don't do. For Hoxter, there is an overlap between the two. However, Hoxter also attests that psychotherapy is concerned primarily with the unconscious and 'deeper disturbances', whereas counselling's focus is on the conscious. By inference, Hoxter is downgrading counselling to dealing with relatively superficial human strife.

The American Counseling Association tries its best to deliver a lucid designation of its business. But its definition of 'professional counseling' is, however, so all-embracing as to be meaningless, tautological (that is, repetitive) and teleological (circular). Nor does it mention psychotherapy or science:

> The application of mental health, psychological, or human development principles, through cognitive, affective, behavioral or systematic intervention strategies, that address wellness, personal growth, or career development, as well as pathology.
>
> (American Counseling Association 2007)

Moreover, this definition by the American Counseling Association was formulated originally in 1997. In the intervening time much has occurred in the therapy world that might have necessitated a definitional refurbishment.

The United Kingdom Council for Psychotherapy goes in for haziness when answering the question (within its 'Frequently Asked Questions' section on its website) 'What is the difference between counselling and psychotherapy?': 'There are many similarities between these disciplines. It is very hard to explain the differences between them' (United Kingdom Council for Psychotherapy 2007). The difference between psychotherapy and counselling does not seem to be set out clearly or steadfastly by therapy practitioners or agencies. For example, the type of client does not provide the basis for separating the two. Both psychotherapists and counsellors work with individuals, groups, families, couples, children, the young, adults and the elderly, and gay, lesbian, trans-sexual, and straight people. Nor are distinct forms of psychological distress the criterion, as both cover problems with relationships; alcohol and drugs; sex; bereavement; 'stress' and misery. Nor does the mode of interaction differ between the therapist and the client (both use predominantly face-to-face contact, but either could use telephone and email or internet methods although these tend to be favoured more by counsellors).

Furthermore, both psychotherapists and counsellors are at liberty to indulge in their personal style of therapy. That is, they do not have to stick to style nominated as 'psychotherapy' or 'counselling'. Their training heritage and any organizational registration/membership requirements may guide their choice, and there is an assumed bias towards short-term therapeutic input by counsellors (especially when psychotherapy is associated with psychoanalytic/dynamic approaches). But either can select from rational-emotive,[3] personal-construct, brief-dynamic, and solution-focused therapies, gestalt, feminism, and constructionism. Or they can choose to combine therapeutic styles (consistently or erratically), and declare themselves as 'eclectic' or 'intergrationalist'.

The NHS Direct Online Health Encyclopaedia uses an all-encompassing description of psychotherapy:

> Psychotherapy is a set of techniques used to treat mental health and emotional problems and some psychiatric disorders. It helps the person to understand and accept their strengths and weaknesses, as well as what makes them feel positive or anxious. Identifying feelings and ways of thinking helps the person to cope with situations they find difficult, and new ways of approaching them.
>
> Psychotherapy is often used to deal with psychological problems that have built up over a number of years. This requires a trusting relationship between the person and the psychotherapist, and treatment usually lasts for months or sometimes years.
>
> (NHS Direct Online Health Encyclopaedia 2007)

So expansive is this portrayal of psychotherapy it could be interpreted as covering a large proportion of human performance, much of which does not need professional intervention (that is, it doesn't distinguish between therapy and the lay and everyday intervention of 'befriending'). Moreover, the aspects of psychological distress referred to are not solely the province of psychotherapy (or counselling). Psychiatrists, general practitioners, clinical psychologists, psychiatric nurses, social workers, and a whole host of other workers and volunteers engaged in the mental health field, have an input into 'emotional problems' and 'psychiatric disorders'.

Hence, this definition of psychotherapy given by the NHS Direct Online Health Encyclopaedia is meaningless. However, an alternative tack to that of the 'broad brush' is taken to depict counselling. Here the NHS Direct Online Health Encyclopaedia offers what it terms as a 'service' description. Oddly, an example provided of a counselling approach is then labelled as a psychotherapy. What is even wackier, however, is that there is a clear statement by the Encyclopaedia about counselling being conducted by a 'trained and independent' person, but reference is made to therapies which do not involve a therapist at all (the client helps him/herself):

There are several types of counselling, or 'talking treatments'. These include:

- Cognitive behavioural therapy (CBT), which retrains our way of thinking to help us deal with stressful situations. This is a form of psychotherapy.
- Self-help (manuals, books, audio tapes, etc.), support groups, and helping.

Counselling is guided discussion with an independent trained person, to help you find your own answers to a problem or issue.
(NHS Direct Online Health Encyclopaedia 2007)

Then there is the Psychotherapy and Counselling Federation of Australia's definition of psychotherapy and counselling. To begin with, this organization states that 'professional' psychotherapists and counsellors are such because they are very well trained, have a contract with the client, and are principled in their dealings with the client. It is the task of trained, contracted and principled counsellors and psychotherapists, states the Federation, to enable: 'individuals to obtain assistance in exploring and resolving issues of an interpersonal, intrapsychic, or personal nature' (The Psychotherapy and Counselling Federation of Australia 2007). So, either the (trained, contracted, and principled) psychotherapist or counsellor can assist an individual with the difficulty he/she has with him/herself or with other people. However, it is not obvious what could possibly separate 'interpersonal and intrapsychic' from 'personal' issues (or private troubles). That is, how could issues in an individual's psyche or the relationships he/she has with others not be 'personal'? Moreover, the organization contradicts the common assumption that psychotherapy is prolonged compared with counselling, but then draws attention to a distinction:

> The work with clients may be of considerable depth in both modalities; however, the focus of Counselling is more likely to be on specific problems or changes in life adjustment. Psychotherapy is more concerned with the restructuring of the personality or self.
> (The Psychotherapy and Counselling Federation of Australia 2007)

But the two statements are not compatible. If both psychotherapy *and* counselling are involved with all things personal, including the 'intrapsychic', how can one be more interested than the other in the 'personality' (or the 'self')? The personality (or the self) is *part* of the individual's intrapsychic constitution.

Conflict, therefore, is manifest at the interface of psychotherapy and counselling, an interface that may not in any case have any substance. A good deal of this friction has arisen because of the history of therapy. However, conflict in therapy is dynamic. Superimposed on the entrenched disputes, are contemporary fragmentations and formation of fiefdoms.

For example, splits have become apparent within psychology, the core 'feeder' discipline for therapy (Bem and de Jong 2006). To begin with, there is the divide between 'pop' or folk psychology and the academic version. Then there is the argument about whether or not psychology is a science, and, if so, what kind of science. American academic psychology leans more towards quantitative measurement and research than its more qualitatively-orientated British counterpart (although, in recent decades there has been a lurch by British psychology towards the quantitative side). Moreover, although there have always been different psychology 'camps', the discipline of psychology could now be disintegrating, with numerous 'psychologies' (such as neo-evolutionary, cognitive, and humanistic) arising from the melee. This would undoubtedly have salient effects on the enterprise of therapy.

Lottery

Such a dramatic renovation of psychology aside, the key strain in the enterprise of therapy is over the explosion in different types of therapy and unremitting swelling of the ranks of therapists. There are hundreds of forms of therapy, ranging across the alphabet from 'acceptance-commitment therapy' to 'vegetotherapy'. But many are what psychologist Margaret Singer and sociologist Janja Lalich (1996) call 'crazy therapies' (and by inference, these are practised by crazy therapists). Moreover, Singer and Lalich made that comment many years ago, and the list has expanded exponentially since that time, incorporating yet more approaches of doubtful therapeutic merit. Journalist Sam Wollaston comments on a television programme about hypochondria. Psychological treatments for the condition are discussed in the programme, and Wollaston decides to try 'balloon therapy' (not the techniques by the same name used to control either menstruation or sinusitis, but one aimed at bursting psychological distress):

> You write something on a balloon you don't like about yourself, then pop the balloon, and it all goes away. I'm going to give it a go. I've written "I'm poor" on a balloon, here's a pin, pop! Now check my bank balance ... I'm still poor. Rubbish, it doesn't work.
>
> (Wollaston 2007)

But fashion and expediency mean that some sane and crazy therapies become more popular than others and then fade away, possibly rediscovered at a later date and given a new lease of life.

However, the fragmentation of the therapeutic enterprise into hundreds of therapies as an indication of disharmony could be construed as misleading. That is, the enterprise can be regarded not to be as complicated or as abundant as at first it would seem because therapies are rooted in one of three core theoretical frameworks. These are psychoanalysis/psychodynamics, humanism, and cognitive-behaviourism. But, use of these three rubrics to subsume most therapies still does need clarification.

Psychoanalysis/psychodynamics

To take the first of these rubrics, psychodynamic theory is the progeny of psychoanalytic theory, albeit a rebellious one. There is much shared theoretical ground to warrant psychoanalytical and psychodynamic theories being referred to conjointly, and they are regularly used as synonyms. But distinctions can be made. These distinctions have arisen from the early acrimonies involving Freud and his collaborators-turned-detractors along with some disloyal post-Freudians, and later as a natural consequence of further insights into the psychology of the psyche along with the need to become more 'efficient' and 'evidential'.

Both psychoanalytical and psychodynamic theorists believe in the existence and influence of the unconscious. Both regard childhood as the most important stage in life that shapes subsequent performance. It is the psychoanalytic/psychodynamic therapist's task is to try to uncover unconscious motivations that stem from unresolved early-life happenings. These unresolved experiences are thought, so psychoanalytic/psychodynamic theorists maintain, to cause psychological distress in later life. To uncover and repair these experiences (using such techniques as 'free association', and the interpretation of dreams, slips of the tongue, symbols, and 'phantasies') could take years if not decades.

But despite the importance paid by both to rummaging around in the unconscious, it was the difference in emphasis of the effect of the unconscious on behaviour, and its relationship to other parts of the psyche and to the external environment, that caused the original rift. Moreover, just how much rummaging can be indulged may depend on whether or not the therapist is purely 'analytical' or merely 'dynamic'. That is, psychodynamic therapy is commonly less protracted compared to psychoanalysis. There are, for example, designated 'short-term' variations of psychodynamic therapy (such as 'brief dynamic therapy', and 'accelerated experiential dynamic therapy'[4]). No doubt the 'brief' and 'accelerated' therapists have sophisticated archaeological implements to enable them to dig into the unconscious as deeply as their more laboured psychodynamic counterparts to excavate 'conserved psychic energy'. But perhaps they do it much faster, or they judiciously cherry-pick what bothers the client most. Therefore, borrowing a marketing term from the food-and-drinks industry, psychodynamic therapy can be described as 'lite' analysis. But, just as 'lite' cola drinks (or yoghurt, baked beans, and mayonnaise) may contain artificial substitutes for the removed 'heavy' ingredients, so psychodynamic therapy can be accused of not being as satisfying as (borrowing the famous cola slogan) the 'real thing'.

Apart from the supposed higher degree of introspection perpetrated in psychodynamics, the client's encounter may not be dissimilar to alternative 'brief' or 'accelerated' therapeutic styles. Furthermore, in both psychoanalytic and psychodynamic therapy a good rapport between therapist and client is considered imperative, as it is (usually) in other forms of therapy. However, there are particular aspects of the relationship that are professed to differentiate psychoanalytic and psychodynamic therapy from the rest. Take notions of 'transference' (the client transfers to the therapist emotions that are associated with another person from the client's life) and 'counter-transference' (the therapist transfers to the client emotions associated with another person from the therapist's life). These were 'invented' by the psychoanalysts, and are considered focal points in both psychoanalytic and psychodynamic practice. But the concepts of transference and counter-transference are now also deliberately used in many other therapies. From Jungian therapy to hypnotherapy, they are either applied to enlighten or enhance the client–therapist relationship, or to illuminate debilitating dependency (Bates 2006).

Moreover, psychodynamic therapy holds key the qualities of empathy, trust, genuineness, and honesty, much more than psychodynamics. But these qualities, originating from humanistic therapy, have been adopted in most types of therapy. It would be therefore inconceivable to have a relationship in *any* therapy founded blatantly on insensitivity, suspicion, pretension, and duplicity.[5]

The intentional or accidental blurring of therapeutic styles is much more probable if a therapist has trained in a number of approaches. The doubly-accredited/registered Principal Psychotherapist and counsellor at 'Harley Therapy' in (*the* Harley Street, famed for private medicine) London, is such a multi-qualified therapist. On the Harley Therapy website (2008), Sheri Jacobson states that she holds seven therapy qualifications. Her credentials cover psychoanalysis, psychodynamics, cognitive-behaviourism, existenti-alism, and humanism. She also holds post-graduate qualifications in social anthropology and philosophy, politics, and economics, and contributes to discussion about a range of psychological topics in the media (for example, friendships for wealthy people, single mothers and sons, battered men, the 'male crisis', positive psychology, and finding love). I'm sure that Dr. Jacobson is mindful during therapy of the genesis of her therapeutic insights, and is capable of either keeping within the particular paradigm, or forms, from her vast theoretical profile, a therapeutically valuable compilation of understandings. However, on the face of it, there should be immense difficulty in pooling the disparate discernments about psychological distress from such an impressive professional and academic pedigree.

Although Spinelli (1994) for one accepts that most therapies can be subsumed under psychoanalysis/psychodynamics, humanism, and cognitive-behaviourism, he does admit that the three rubrics are not complementary. It is as if such seemingly irreconcilable treatments for cancer as the excision of the offending tumour, wafting herbs over it, and dancing around virgins in the dead of night to stimulate mystical intervention, have been legitimized. The surgeons, herbalists, and occultists may all be trying to accomplish the same end (curing the cancer), but the way to reach that end varies considerably. Moreover, excision and wafting have the advantage of swiftness and social acceptability compared with enacting ritualistic rhythms – let alone the difficulty in procuring virgins.

Oh, yes, just to add further sludge to the already muddied waters of the therapeutic enterprise, not only is there psychoanalytic/psychodynamic psychotherapy, but there is also psychoanalytic/psychodynamic counselling! Hence, a possible distinction between psychotherapy and counselling on the basis of length and depth disintegrates when the arch proponents of length and depth migrate to the 'short' and 'superficial' camp. Just to complete the murky hydro analogy, there is also humanistic counselling and humanistic psychotherapy, cognitive-behavioural therapy, cognitive-behavioural psychotherapy, and cognitive-behavioural counselling.

Humanism

Humanistic therapy, like psychoanalytic/psychodynamic therapy, has its contradictions and tangles. To begin with, 'humanism' is an idiom which is invoked in other fields than therapy. For example, humanism is a political-ethical philosophy which promotes the idea that people have sovereignty over their lives and should be guided by reason, not religion or superstition.

Contrasting the humanism of a political-ethical hue to that of humanistic therapy, there are considerably more political-ethical humanists than there are humanist therapists and their clients. But more significantly sociologically, there are far greater social penalties aimed at, and social responsibilities taken by, the former than the latter.

An example of the social penalty for being a political-ethical humanist is that while there is little or no approbation directed towards secularists (including humanists) in Europe (and 36 per cent of the British population alone count themselves as humanists: British Humanist Association 2007), this is not true elsewhere. But in the USA, where Christian fundamentalism has been revived and being 'theist' (that is, believing in a God) is expected, there is appreciable discrimination against humanists. According to the American Humanist Association (2007), despite millions of US citizens being non-religious (or superstitious), less than 50 per cent of the US population would vote for an atheist presidential candidate. Moreover, admitting being non-theist (as one Congressman did in 2007) is described by the American Humanist Association as akin to 'coming out' as a homosexual. In Muslim countries, particularly those that have adopted Sharia Law, not believing in Islam, whether as a humanist or as a believer in another religion, can lead to subjugation or death (Mirza 2002). It is unlikely that being a humanist therapist or a client of a humanist therapist will induce any fear of punishment, apart from that which is induced by the gruelling task of pulling off self-actualization.

With reference to social responsibility, the American Humanist

Association has joined the 'Save Darfur Coalition'. The Coalition campaigns against the ongoing genocide in the Darfur region of Sudan Darfur. Since 2004, millions of people have either been killed or displaced in a state-orchestrated ethnic conflict, with little international action mustered to prevent its continuation (Morrall 2006a). What the American Humanist Association urges is that the American Government supports the sending of a sizeable multinational military force to protect the civilians of Darfur. It is unlikely that any humanist therapy organization would align itself so decidedly with armed intervention in the affairs of another country.

Furthermore, there is an assortment of humanist therapies. These include: gestalt; transactional analysis; logotherapy; and motivational interviewing. Humanistic principles are also often commandeered by practitioners who are either using other traditions (such as positive psychology), are joining two approaches together (as in 'humanistic-existentialism'; and mosaic-humanistic counselling), or are claiming to be 'eclectic' or 'holistic'.

Carl Rogers' brand of humanistic counselling was first called by him 'client-centred', but later 'person-centred'. This modification would appear to have been made to underscore the humanist belief in personal growth, and empowerment. The label of 'client' implies that there is a social distance between the person and the therapist. But of course that social distance always exists, no matter what appellation is applied. Most clients come to therapy presumably because they believe that therapists have an expertise that they do not have. That expertise may be employed to enhance the personal growth and empowerment of the client by allowing the client to tell his/her story in the way that he/she wishes. Nevertheless, it is the therapist who has studied that method, and has the knowledge, skills, and attitudes to facilitate an outcome that the method regards as fitting.

The qualities of the Rogerian humanist (empathy, trust, genuineness, and honesty) are transferable across therapy practices. But because attention is given to the 'here and now' rather than past events (and certainly does not pander to childhood rummaging), and the conscious not the unconscious, there is an unbridgable chasm that separates Rogerian theory and practice from that derived from Freud. Moreover, psychoanalytical/psychodynamic therapy is rarely practised in either state-run or private health services because of the long-term cost implications and the difficulty of demonstrating that it is effective (given the contemporary measurements employed to support 'evidence-based' health practices). Whilst the qualities of humanism (empathy, trust, genuineness, and honesty) are propagated throughout therapy, unadulterated humanistic therapy is also considered an indulgence in the cost-obsessed world of contemporary health care. However, the third therapeutic rubric *is* indulged.

Cognitive-behaviourism

Cognitive-behavioural therapy became the vogue treatment in many Western countries (for example, the USA, Canada, Britain, Australia, New Zealand, Germany, and France) early in the twenty-first century. Although cognitive-behavioural therapy is an amalgam of behavioural and cognitive psychologies, the two elements have their own therapeutic rationale about human performance. Put simply, behaviourists aren't much bothered about thinking, and cognitivists aren't too concerned with doing. Moreover, the 'behaviour' part of cognitive-behavioural therapy has two roots (classical and operant) which posit divergent notions about human conduct. One drew its knowledge from making dogs salivate through the ringing of bells, and the other from a system of 'reinforcers' and 'eliminators' with rats.

So, cognitive-behavioural therapy attempts to amalgamate psychologies with their conceptual and empirical base inherited from observations of dogs and rats (cats and pigeons also played their part) with the intricate psychological analysis of the reasoning powers of the human mind and neurological functioning. Notwithstanding this momentous intellectual quandary, the avowed intention of the cognitive-behavioural therapist is to promote new ways of thinking by clients about their personal problems in order to manipulate emotions and behaviours. But not any type of thinking will do. Not only have the freshly implanted ruminative blueprints to be relevant to the issue troubling the client and be in the conscious 'here and now', they must be positive. That is, despite the antagonism towards the retrospective-brooding of psychoanalytical/psychodynamic therapy, and an aficionado of objective measurement, the cognitive-behaviourist ultimately slips into subjective judgements about what is good and what is bad for the client.

The antipathy to in-depth and prolonged reflection is both cognitive-behavioural therapy's selling point and its Achilles' heel. It has become popular among the auditors and accountants of health care services because it can furnish changes in human performance relatively quickly, and it can demonstrate that these have taken place.

But as a 'quick fix' approach, cognitive-behavioural therapy is accused of not being substantive enough to maintain those changes. For the British Consultant Psychotherapist and Psychiatrist Jeremy Holmes (2002), cognitive-behavioural therapy's success is more apparent than real. Therapy, he argues, should not be aimed simply at the technical elimination of symptoms or disorders (such as depression, anxiety, or compulsions) because the client's 'development trajectory' needs to be grasped. Moreover, the assessment of any therapy through the 'trials' of the 'medical metaphor' are inadequate as their effectiveness needs to be judged not only in the long term but also in the real world in which the client lives.

Cognitive-behavioural therapy, much more than other therapies, has also been taken up by a host of lay and professional 'helpers'. Specialist registration and accreditation bodies (for example, the 'British Association of Behavioural and Cognitive Psychotherapies'; and in the USA, 'National Association of Cognitive-Behavioral Therapists') set standards for training courses. However, the length and depth of training available internationally vary enormously from one-year full-time master's course run by universities to one-day workshops operated by private companies. Training is also offered by post. For example, the 'Open College' (2007) advertises what it describes as a 'rich and very deep' distance learning diploma programme for therapists, doctors, nurses, lawyers, psychologists, social workers, drug workers, police officers, and shop, office, and factory workers, as well as labourers. The programme lasts 3–6 months. It is supported by a 'highly stimulating course text book', a study-time log, and a free relaxation CD (although it is not clear if the CD is part of learning the therapeutic technique or is to deal with the surfeit of documentary encouragement). Those who successfully complete the diploma, the Open College states, are entitled to use a string of letters ('Dip.CBT MOC & MSFTR') after their name.

A throng of therapists

It is impossible to calculate accurately how many therapists there are in the world because: there is relatively easy access to therapy tuition, and much of it is non-standardized; a surplus of therapies already exists, but there is no control over further inventions (and invention by definition has no benchmark); borders are porous between therapy, the normal work of medical/health and caring occupations, helping, friendship, and advising; the territory of the therapeutic enterprise is being encroached upon by, for example, life-coaches (Williams 2003) and philosophers (LeBon 2001); no accepted accreditation/registration system is *in situ* globally, or even within some countries (with most countries of the world having no system at all).

Stefan Priebe and Donna Wright (2006), however, do provide an insight into the numbers of therapists in few countries. They estimate that there are 38,000 members of counselling/psychotherapy associations in the UK; in the Netherlands there are approximately 5,000 psychotherapists; Russia has about 3,278 state psychotherapists and 6,155 private psychotherapists (psychotherapy is provided by either medically trained psychotherapists or medical psychologists); Switzerland has roughly 1,264 adult psychiatrists and 2,461 psychological psychotherapists (psychotherapists are either psychiatrists or psychologists); Germany has 16,000 psychological psychotherapists and 3,500 medical psychotherapists (psychotherapy is only provided by doctors and some psychologists). Australia has approximately 900 registered psychotherapists and counsellors, 1,000 clinical psychologists, 900 counselling psychologists, and 250 psychiatrists practising psychotherapy.

France, record Priebe and Wright, has between 8,000–12,000 psychotherapists. In 2004, an amendment was made by the French government to an ancient law which was implemented to protect the public from the 'magical doings of Gypsies and cults'. From that date onwards it is only medical practitioners, and clinical psychologists, along with those on a special register who are not doctors or psychologists, who are allowed to carry out therapy (and there is a bias towards psychoanalysis in France). Anyone else dabbling in therapy faces a criminal conviction.

Winners and losers

So, when someone wants to choose a therapist and therapy, how can they choose? At present, it is similar to picking the numbers for a lottery ticket. Perhaps the numbers are picked because they have brought winnings for a friend, relative, or colleague. Maybe, there is a meticulous study of how regular a series of numbers appear. More probably it is the lucky dip of randomness. Just what therapy, and which therapist, is selected from the bewildering range of possibilities comes about from personal recommendation, or reviewing the evidence of which one works. But (especially at a time of psychological distress) far more likely is that either part or the whole of the choice will be made because the therapist is available and accessible, has some letters after his/her name, and the therapy/therapist 'feels right'. Assessment of 'rightness', however, may not be wholly impartial but be contaminated by the inevitable self-serving impulses of the therapy enterprise and the understandable self-deluding wishes of its clientele. Trying to win money this way might be perfectly acceptable (and – allegedly – 'fun'), but not fixing perturbed minds. Being 'wrong' playing the lottery is to be expected given the odds declared by its proprietors against winning a sizeable financial prize. Being 'wrong' playing therapy should *not* be expected given the odds declared by its disciples for substantive psychological success.

Rivalry

It is somewhat tricky for a person who is probably not as discerning as they would be normally (because he/she is in a state of mental turbulence) to choose a therapy and therapist. Selection by proxy might, therefore, be an answer.

A would-be client may already be seeking advice for their psychological distress from his/her general practitioner. Apart from prescribing mind medication, the general practitioner may employ a therapist, or retain a list of recommended private therapists. However, although fictional, David Lodge in his novel *Therapy*, illustrates how there may be a disjunction between what is proposed by the medical practitioner and what is desired by the patient. The main character in the novel, Tubby Passmore, is going through a mid-life crisis as well as inexplicable knee pain. His general practitioner recommends a cognitive-behavioural therapist called Alexandra:

> "She's very good", he [the general practitioner] assured me. "She's very practical. Doesn't waste time poking around in your unconscious, asking about potty training, or whether you saw your parents having it off together, that sort of thing" ... And Alexandra certainly has been a help ... I always feel much calmer after seeing her, for at least a couple of hours ... There are times, through, when I hanker after a bit of old-fashioned Viennese analysis.
>
> (Lodge 1995: 16)

Tubby's hankering is, moreover, laying bare the contemporary tension within the therapeutic enterprise between 'mind-managing' (practical but cursory types of therapy: especially cognitive-behavioural) and 'mind-mining' (impractical but profound types of therapy: specifically analytical/dynamic).

Another proxy technique for obtaining a therapist/therapy is to contact one of the therapy agencies. But this is no guarantee of excellence, and may be a very misleading method of picking a person or a proclivity. To begin with, the agencies of therapy are fragmented and replete with enmity (House 2003; Totton 2006). Hence, whoever and whatever is listed will reflect the inherent rivalries within the therapeutic enterprise, but not necessary overtly so. A prospective client can be blithely unaware that the therapist and therapy he/she is considering is viewed by others in the therapeutic enterprise as at best futile and at worse heinous. Many therapy agencies simply list therapists who pay the membership fee. Others act as registration bodies and demand proof of training and supervision. Some agencies allow impending clients to gain access to their lists to find a therapist, but may not provide detailed curricula vitae (which generally are submitted by the therapists and may not be verified by the agencies). Moreover, most incorporate no aspects of society ('asocial therapy') or only a semblance of social factors ('naïve social therapy'), and are also intensely conservative. Virtually none to date can be classified as 'authentic social therapy', although a few have radical pretensions.

Therapy now traverses the world, from Albania to New Zealand via the Cameroon, and Norway to Uruguay via Iran (Pritz 2002). But the assortment, number, intertwining, claims, personas, proliferation, incongruities, and positioning of therapy agencies are baffling and alarming.

International umbrellas

To begin with, umbrella organizations compete for dominant representation in supra-state or international bodies such as the European Union and the United Nations. The International Association for Counselling (2007) had been the 'The International Round Table for the Advancement of Counselling', but in 1997 decided its pursuance of 'advancement' had been so successful it could be dropped from its title (and presumably sitting around round tables had also had its day). It is recognized by the United Nations Educational, Scientific and Cultural Organization as a non-governmental organization, and has official consultative status with the Council of Europe. Below are the agencies affiliated to the International Association for Counselling:

- Academy of Certified Counsellors
- African Counselling Network
- All Russian Psychotherapeutic League
- American Counseling Association
- American School Counsellor Association
- Asociación Argentina de Counselors
- Associação Portuguesa de Psicoterapia Centrada na Pessoa e de Counselling (Portugal)
- Association des Conseillers d'Orientation – Psychologues (France)
- Association for Family Therapy and Systemic Practice in the UK
- Association française de counseling dans l'approche centrée sur la personne (France)
- Australian Association of Career Counsellors
- Australian Counselling Association
- Australian Guidance and Counselling Association
- British Association for Counselling and Psychotherapy

- British Association for Sexual and Relationship Therapy
- Canadian Counselling Association
- Centro Risorse Europeo per l'Orientamento (European Resource Centre for Guidance)
- Council for Accreditation of Counselling and Related Educational Programs
- Counselling in Nederland
- Counsellors and Psychotherapists Association of New South Wales (CAPA)
- Danish National Council for Educational and Vocational Guidance
- Federación Española de Asociaciones de Psicoterapeutas (Spain)
- Holos-San Isidro (Argentina)
- Institute of Careers Guidance
- Institute of Guidance Counsellors
- International Association for Educational and Vocational Guidance
- International Association of Counseling Services
- International Counseling Network
- International Federation for Psychotherapy
- International Institute of Psychosomatic Medicine
- International Society of Professional Counsellors
- Irish Association for Counselling and Therapy
- National Board of Certified Counsellors and Affiliates
- National Centre for Guidance in Education
- New Zealand Association of Counsellors
- Singapore Association for Counselling
- Società Italiana di Counseling (Italy)

Then there is the World Council for Psychotherapy (2007), with its commendably impressive purpose: to unite all therapists, and all therapeutic national and international agencies, *everywhere*. But, despite being a nongovernmental organization of the United Nation's Economic and Social Council, its avowed loyalty is to the *European*-orientated 'Strasbourg Declaration on Psychotherapy of 1990'. Moreover, in 2007, the World Council for Psychotherapy announced that it would be able 'without any problems' to award a '*World* Certificate for Psychotherapy' to anyone who had earned the *European* Certificate for Psychotherapy from the *European* Association for Psychotherapy (on payment to one or the other of 350 Euros).

The European Association for Psychotherapy, which started certificate-awarding ten years prior to the World Council for Psychotherapy, represents 128 therapy agencies (26 of which are national umbrella organizations and 18 are European associations for psychotherapy) from 41 European countries. It has a membership of more than 120,000 therapists. A significant element of the Strasbourg Declaration on Psychotherapy of 1990 is the description of therapy as *scientific*. The World Council for Psychotherapy endorses this view of therapy. For example, it describes therapy as a 'human *science*'. It is interesting then to find that the World Council for Psychotherapy has a *spirituality* section. Moreover, another inconsistency arises in the World Council for Psychotherapy and the European Association for Psychotherapy's stance on therapy as science. They do not exclude from awarding their respective certificates to therapists who gain qualifications in countries (such as Britain) where training is largely non-scientific, pseudo-scientific, or quasi-scientific.

Beside the general umbrella therapy agencies, there are specialist umbrella therapy agencies. The International Psychoanalytical Association (2007) claims not only to be the largest worldwide agency representing psychoanalysis, but also the primary accrediting and regulatory body for psychoanalysts. It has 11,500 members from 33 countries, and dozens of constituent organizations:

- Australian Psychoanalytical Society
- Belgian Psychoanalytic Society
- Belgrade Psychoanalytical Society
- British Psychoanalytic Association
- British Psychoanalytical Society
- Czech Psychoanalytical Society
- Danish Psychoanalytical Society
- Dutch Psychoanalytical Association
- Dutch Psychoanalytical Group
- Dutch Psychoanalytical Society
- Finnish Psychoanalytical Society
- French Psychoanalytical Association
- German Psychoanalytical Association
- German Psychoanalytical Society
- Hellenic Psychoanalytical Society
- Hungarian Psychoanalytical Society
- Indian Psychoanalytical Society
- Israel Psychoanalytic Society
- Italian Psychoanalytical Association
- Italian Psychoanalytical Society
- Madrid Psychoanalytical Association
- Norwegian Psychoanalytical Society

- Paris Psychoanalytical Society
- Polish Psychoanalytical Society
- Portuguese Psychoanalytical Society
- Spanish Psychoanalytical Society
- Swedish Psychoanalytical Association
- Swedish Psychoanalytical Society
- Swiss Psychoanalytical Society
- Viennese Psychoanalytical Society
- Argentine Psychoanalytic Association
- Argentine Psychoanalytic Society
- Brasília Psychoanalytic Society
- Brazilian Psychoanalytical Society of Porto Alegre
- Brazilian Psychoanalytical Society of Ribeirão Preto
- Brazilian Psychoanalytic Society of Rio de Janeiro
- Brazilian Psychoanalytic Society of São Paulo
- Buenos Aires Psychoanalytic Association
- Caracas Psychoanalytic Society
- Chilean Psychoanalytic Association
- Colombian Psychoanalytic Association
- Colombian Psychoanalytic Society
- Córdoba Psychoanalytic Society
- Freudian Psychoanalytical Society of Colombia
- Mato Grosso do Sul Psychoanalytical Society
- Mendoza Psychoanalytic Society
- Mexican Association for Psychoanalytic Practice, Training and Research
- Mexican Psychoanalytic Association
- Monterrey Psychoanalytic Association
- Pelotas Psychoanalytic Society
- Peru Psychoanalytic Society
- Porto Alegre Psychoanalytic Society
- Psychoanalytical Association of The State of Rio De Janeiro – Rio IV
- Psychoanalytic Society of Mexico – Park Mexico
- Recife Psychoanalytic Society
- Rio de Janeiro Psychoanalytic Society
- Rio III Psychoanalytic Association
- Rosario Psychoanalytic Association
- Uruguayan Psychoanalytical Association
- Venezuelan Psychoanalytic Association
- North America including Japan
- American Psychoanalytic Association
- Canadian Psychoanalytic Society

- Institute for Psychoanalytic Studies
- Institute for Psychoanalytic Training and Research
- Japan Psychoanalytic Society
- Los Angeles Institute and Society for Psychoanalytic Studies
- New York Freudian Society
- Northwestern Psychoanalytic Society
- Psychoanalytic Center of California
- Psychoanalytic Institute of Northern California

Some of these agencies are classified mysteriously as 'provisional' or 'interim provisional'. Others not included in the above inventory are described puzzlingly as 'study groups' (for example: the Croatian Psycho-analytical Study Group; the Guadalajara Psychoanalytic Study Group; the Moscow Psychoanalytic Society Study Group; and the Turkish Psycho-analytical Study Group). One stands on its own under the heading 'guest study group' (the Korean Psychoanalytical Society).

The International Psychoanalytical Association (2007) states that its intention is the establishment of a psychoanalytic 'scientific society', and all of the members of this society will have reached 'exacting standards'. Given the array of agencies (and in some cases multiple agencies from one country) and therefore training programmes, this seems yet another laud-able yet highly ambitious goal emanating from an umbrella therapy agency.

National umbrellas

Representational lucidity and harmony appear no better when comparing national situation or the circumstances within a country than it is globally. Take as examples Australia, the USA, and Britain.

The Psychotherapy and Counselling Federation of Australia (2007) is a national umbrella agency which encompasses the following inventory of agencies:

- Australian Counselling Association
- Australian Board of Certified Counsellors
- Association of Personal Counsellors
- Association of Solution Oriented Counsellors and Hypnotherapists of Australia
- Association of Soul Centred Psychotherapists Inc
- Australian Association of Group Psychotherapists
- Australian and New Zealand Association of Psychotherapy (NSW Branch)
- Australian and New Zealand Psychodrama Association

- Australian and New Zealand Society of Jungian Analysts
- Australian Association of Marriage and Family Counsellors
- Australian Association of Somatic Psychotherapists
- Australian Association of Spiritual Care and Pastoral Counselling
- Australian National Art Therapy Association
- Australian Hypnotherapists Association
- Australian Radix Bodycentred Psychotherapy Association
- Australian Somatic Integration Association
- Christian Counsellors Association
- Clinical Counsellors Association
- Counselling and Psychotherapy Association Canberra and Region
- Counselling Association of South Australia
- Counsellors and Psychotherapists Association of Canberra and Region
- Counsellors and Psychotherapists Association of NSW
- Counsellors and Psychotherapists Association of Victoria
- Dance Therapy Association of Australia
- Emotional Release Counsellors Association of NSW
- Gestalt Australia and New Zealand
- Music and Imagery Association of Australia
- New South Wales Family Therapy Association
- Professional Counsellors Association of Tasmania
- Psychoanalytic Psychotherapy Association of Australasia
- Psychotherapists and Counsellors Association of WA
- Queensland Association for Family Therapy
- Queensland Counsellors Association
- Queensland Transpersonal and Emotional Release Counsellors Association
- Victorian Association of Family Therapists
- Victorian Child Psychotherapists Association
- Western Pacific Association of Transactional Analysis

Apart from not being truly 'national' (some of its member agencies traverse Australia *and* New Zealand), whatever rules and values the Psychotherapy and Counselling Federation of Australia extols, they are not supported by government regulations. Politically, Australia is federalized. As a consequence registration is not regulated nationally. PsychOz (2007), an Australian-based therapy resource website, points out that not only are there many boards to which therapists can apply to register across the country, but training is very dispersed (courses are offered by state and territory tertiary institutions, professional associations, and private institutes). The Australian (federal) Government has moved away from taking responsibility for the regulation of therapists, wanting self-regulation to be installed by therapy agencies (Priebe and Wright 2006). Furthermore, the only (federal) government legislation relevant to therapy in Australia relates to the use of the title 'psychologist'. By law, anyone working as a psychologist has to be registered (the requirements for registration determined by the Psychologists Registration Board of each state and territory).

A similar set-up for therapy (and psychology) as Australia occurs in the USA, and to a large extent for the same reasons – that is, its federal political structure, and lack of willingness by the Federal Government to take on the overall responsibility for regulation. The American Counseling Association (2007) asserts that it is the world's largest association (45,000 members) for 'professional' counsellors, and offers the 'best professional liability insurance program in the industry'. Although its title might suggest otherwise, it recruits not just from the USA but from 50 other countries (Europe, Latin America, the Philippines, and the Virgin Islands). Internet continuing-education courses of 'high-quality' and 'low-cost' are obtainable through the American Counseling Association. Some examples are: Herbaceuticals (an overview for Counselors); Play and Humor in Counseling; Use of Spiritual and Religious Beliefs in Pursuit of Client's Goals; Cybercounseling: Going the Distance for Your Clients.

The American Psychotherapy Association (2007) has about 3,000 members, and it offers therapy credentials, standards, identity, and self-regulation for professional psychotherapists. It states that its purpose is to establish a cohesive national agency for its 'ethical, highly-educated and well-trained' members, and to improve the public perception of therapy (which it enticingly but without elaboration claims has in the USA become devalued in recent years by insurance companies, the court system, and other professional membership associations). Given that commendable goal, it is odd that it provides the following rider:

> The American Psychotherapy Association (APA) does not endorse, guarantee, or warrant the credentials, work, or opinions of any individual member. Membership in APA does not constitute the grant of a license or other licensing authority by or on behalf of the organization as to a member's qualifications, abilities, or expertise.
>
> (American Psychotherapy Association 2007)

British governments, with fluctuating support from the main therapy agencies, have been trying to set up national regulations for therapists since the 1970s. The British Government presently (2007) is embarked on a determined drive to have a statutory monitoring role for therapists, with the implication that the Health Professions Council of the Department of Health will take on this function.

In Britain, there are about 3,8000 members of 34 therapy agencies. There are no mandatory membership requirements, or routes of entry to training, and nearly 600 different training courses (Priebe and Wright 2006). There is also an unknown number of therapists working without any organizational affiliation. Three main (in terms of numbers of members) national umbrella agencies operate in Britain. The British Association for Counselling (2007), the largest of the three (with 24,000 members[6]) was founded in the 1970s from voluntary sector groups. By 2000, it had changed its name to incorporate 'psychotherapy', becoming the British Association for Counselling and Psychotherapy. This, it proclaimed, was in acknowledgement of counsellors and psychotherapists wanting to belong to a united profession. Representation and registration of psychotherapists had already been taking place in Britain since 1993 by the second largest agency, the United Kingdom Council for Psychotherapy (2007). It has about 6,200 members and incorporates approximately 80 therapy organizations (including some with loyalty to counselling rather than psychotherapy). These organizations tender a multiplicity of therapy modes.

But, and this is a problem for many, if not all, umbrella agencies, such a wide encompassment of styles results in both complementary and incompatible therapies being lumped together. This poses a considerable impediment in terms of representation and the setting of standards. How can a united voice and similar practice principles be formulated for hypnosis, autogenic therapy, neuro-linguistic programming, and women's therapy (all of which are embraced by the United Kingdom Council for Psychotherapy)? Moreover, the United Kingdom Council for Psychotherapy's list of member organizations incorporates those with a psychodynamic/psychoanalytical bent (for example, the Confederation for Analytical Psychology, and the Centre for Freudian Analysis and Research). Again, this throws up a hitch concerning representation and standards which is shared with other umbrella agencies. That is, there is a major contender, and in this case it is the third largest therapy agency in Britain: The British Psychoanalytic Council. With roughly 1,200 members (deemed as 'registrants'), The British Psychoanalytic Council (2007) claims that it is the 'leading voice' for the psychodynamic/psychoanalytic sector of therapy. Member Organisations of Council are:

- British Association of Psychotherapists
- British Psychoanalytical Society
- Lincoln Clinic and Centre for Psychotherapy

- London Centre for Psychotherapy
- North of England Association for Training in Psychoanalytic Psychotherapy
- Northern Ireland Association for the Study of Psychoanalysis
- Scottish Association of Psychoanalytical Psychotherapists
- Scottish Institute of Human Relations
- Severnside Institute for Psychotherapy
- Society of Analytical Psychology
- Tavistock Clinic and Tavistock Society of Psychotherapists
- Association for Psychoanalytic Psychotherapy in the NHS

The affirmed profile of the British Psychoanalytic membership, however, is unusual for an umbrella therapy agency, and could be considered an historical hangover from the elitist genesis of therapy. The British Psychoanalytic Council states that many of its members are leading figures in the field of mental health (for example, senior consultant psychiatrists and clinical psychologists).

Social therapy

Whereas Freud was most definitely a radical (and his legacy continues to cause trouble today), it is doubtful whether today's 'leading figures in the field of mental health' are likely to rebel against the social system and health service that employs them and to which they are accountable. Freud's thinking and practice were way 'outside the box', drastically innovative, and emphatically disturbing to late-nineteenth-century and early twentieth-century society. But the present internal muddles and struggles of the therapeutic enterprise, along with its enduring deliberation on the microcosm of human suffering, have turned it into yet another one of the problems of the world, not a solution to the problems of the world. Such indulgencies detract from the black hole of global human despair and endemic ecological catastrophe.

Michael Bennett (2004), attempting to answer the question 'what is the purpose of therapy?', argues that while socially philanthropic pledges have been avowed, these have been sacrificed for more narcissistic goals (for example, the drive to gain professional status). However, recognition that there is such a thing as society does surface occasionally. Some therapists serendipitously respond to the impact of social factors on their clients (for example, by referring to the positive and negative bearing of significant others on his/her life). Some therapies candidly give credence to influences external to the individual (such as his/her family).

Therapies orientated to 'the social' in one guise or another have been practised since the middle of the twentieth century. For example, the British psychiatrist David Clark (1974) introduced 'social therapy' into psychiatric institutions. He believed that for long-term psychiatric patients the 'therapeutic community' (a concept that had been developed by army psychiatrists and psychoanalysts in the 1940s) became more of an appropriate 'treatment' than medication. Staff of the institution and patients would work together to resolve personal, interpersonal, and community issues/troubles, and find a way of living together conducive to mental health.

Parallel disciplines to therapy may also reflect on society. For example, Critical Psychology International (2007) was formed in 2003. It is a network of psychologists who wish to have more understanding of how social factors affect mental health introduced into mainstream psychology. Originating in 1993, the Radical Psychology Network (2007) also wants to revise mainstream psychology and alter society's status quo. It has the aim of bringing about a better world through social justice and reform. Critical Psychiatry Network consists of psychiatrists and other workers in the mental health who want to see a shift towards social approaches. They criticize the dominance of neuroscience as an explanatory framework for mental disorder and pharmaceutical treatments.

A number of therapy organizations (for example, the Psychotherapy and Counselling Federation of Australia; the American Counseling Association; World Council for Psychotherapy) do refer to social policies in their missions or make direct contributions to debates about public issues. The British relationship therapy service *Relate* (2008b), has specific information on 'relationships and society'. Reference is made to the links between unstable families, and social problems such as poverty and homelessness.

But this is what I term 'naïve social therapy'. Socially aware therapists, therapies, and therapy agencies do rival the foremost (conservative) impulse of the therapeutic enterprise. But this is not to the degree that propels substantive social change. Such rival positioning only touches the surface of social determinants of human performance and offers merely tokenistic challenges to the social system. Moreover, it is dismissed or ignored by most politicians, most grandees of the therapeutic enterprise, and most therapists.

However, some therapists *do* propose more 'authentic social therapy'. These few radicals *are* raising their sights from the circumscribed navel-gazing of therapy, seeing above the parapet of self-indulgence, and argue for social responsibility and social action to be an integral part of the therapeutic enterprise. Authentic social therapy goes beyond the individual's interpersonal connections and the gates of her/his institutional allegiances to recognize the dynamics of global society.

Group therapy is typically the coming together of individuals to learn about appropriate social performance from each other and is therefore hardly revolutionary. However, some group therapies have been transformed into politically active 'social therapy' by embracing particular sociological perspectives such as postmodernism or Marxism (Holzman and Mendez 2003; Newman and Holzman 2000).

An international team of therapy theorists and practitioners claim that the 'person-centred' is 'political' because of its commitment to the emancipation of humanity (Proctor et al. 2006). Person-centred therapy regards all clients as inherently decent and having an essential ability to change their lives. Such an outlook on the human condition becomes a political position about the power of individuals to improve society. Proctor et al. argue that person-centred therapy can foment social change (by which they mean, for example, the reawakening of grass-roots democracy; respect for the elderly; an increase in public safety and decline in warfare; an acceptance of diversity; environmental conservation; and sustainable economics). For them, an outcome of the person-centred therapeutic relationship needs to be combined with person-centred politics whereby therapists 'speak with one voice'.

Summary

Mark Burton (2004) refers to the 'postmodern' virus that affects the work of some of the radical psychology organizations. Thus, he argues that the problem with postmodernism is that social reality is not accepted as ever being real (that is, there are many realities, all of which are equally valid), and what is not taken into account is that structural reform is necessary to improve society. This criticism I suggest can also be levelled at many of the radical therapy agencies, along with the criticism that 'speaking with one voice' is not remotely possible when therapy is such a lottery, and so filled with conflict and rivalry, thereby a profoundly troubled discipline. Human suffering is real and real social change demands the structure of society to be transformed radically.

The philosopher and psychoanalyst, George Frankl (2000; 2003; 2004), links culture with consciousness and society with psychological distress. What Frankl argues is that the diminution or implausibility of moral directives from governments results in mental disorder and anti-social behaviour. That is, unconsciously humans are struggling with the moral void and/or contradictions that characterize Western civilization (but which are spreading fast globally). For Frankl, such inner torment leads to neuroses and psychoses.

David Smail (1999; 2001; 2006) points out that society is structured by compelling influences, which individuals cannot surmount. Consequently, for much of the time people do not have a choice. Therapists of all persuasions (psychoanalytical, humanist, and especially cognitive-behavioural), claims Smail, are therefore misleading clients, and he wonders why, given the obviousness of social constraints over individual freedom and responsibility for human performance.

Nick Totton (2000) observes therapy has for over the century of its existence been constantly interacting with politics at both the micro and macro level. If Totton's observation is correct, such a long-standing association has had precious little influence, given the state of global society. Smail concludes that it is not in the interests of therapists and their agencies to pay too much attention to the socially generated limitations on personal liberty. The therapeutic enterprise needs to individualize social problems and encourage clients to believe they can alter their lives because otherwise 'cure' becomes the responsibility of politicians not therapists. Put starkly, the therapeutic enterprise would go out of business if it did not sponsor individualism.

So the social contexts of Heather's childhood and adulthood are supposed, through therapy, to be reinterpretable, manageable, and conquerable. The social changes in her history and social pressures in her present can be therapeutically compartmentalized or dismissed. Psychological stability, and possibly psychological excellence, can be achieved in the face of ill-defined and contrary role expectations (motherhood; employment; marriage), and financial realities (paying for health, housing, transport, schooling, and holidays). In a disordered and disintegrating global society the individual can triumph is the message from therapy, and personal quandaries (including those of Heather) can be re-routed along a single track to a calmer destination.

CHAPTER 3

Arrogant

Science
Scientization
Fallacy

Virginia Ironside, journalist and previous regular client of therapy, who has turned into one of its most vehement critics, is in little doubt: 'Counselling and therapy is surely more of a religion, a faith, than a science' (Ironside, in Bates 2006: 119). For such 'therapy survivors' as Ironside, there is an insufferable self-serving and self-validating arrogance that oozes from the enterprise of therapy. Medical practitioners are professionally arrogant. The history of occupational advancement for medicine has been built on mystifying what it is capable of doing or not doing so that patients' 'faith' in doctors is affirmed. That faith in the doctor as an individual has been replaced by a faith in (medical) science. But unlike unadulterated faith, medical science does seem to provide solutions to some human physical and psychological problems, and so the arrogance of medicine, although irritating, can be regarded as justified. The enterprise of therapy, on the other hand, is struggling to demonstrate efficacy. Its arrogance is more based on insecurity.

Our 'client', Heather, is also arrogant. Her intellect, wit, and demeanour give her the means by which her aloofness is conveyed to, and impressively disarms, her perceived antagonists. On first meeting she gives off a conspicuous aura of self-belief and self-solidity. However, as with the enterprise of therapy, this is a smokescreen. Heather is implausibly unsure of her 'self' and improbably scared of losing the respect of others. She, sometimes consciously, and at other times unconsciously, uses aloofness and condescension to hide her deep-rooted terror of failure and entrenched inability to handle criticism.

Arrogance permeates virtually every nook and cranny of the therapy process. It starts with the inherent disdain for the client's disempowered state when asking for help. Presumably, the client on entering therapy is in a condition of emotional turmoil, unable to think clearly about past and present events in his/her personal life, let alone plan objectively. Otherwise why is he/she bothering with therapy? Notwithstanding the 'therapy junkies' (clients who become dependent on or addicted to therapy, and therapists who become dependent on or addicted to its rewards), most people do not know precisely what to expect from therapy. Even if they do have inklings about how the practice elements of the therapeutic enterprise work, they are likely to be 'passive' in the client–therapist relationship and the therapist 'active'.[1] That is, the therapist, with his/her training and experiences, already has a framework within which he/she operates. This pre-given *modus operandi* may confer rules, originating from a particular therapeutic approach, about calculating effectiveness. So the client might do most of the talking, but the talk is located and interpreted through a prejudicial frame chosen by the therapist as are the measures of therapeutic success or failure.

For example, if the approach is psychoanalytical/dynamic, then uncovering childhood incidents that seem to connect with adult problems could be regarded as a triumphant upshot of the therapy. A client who dispenses with the services of the humanist, declaring that he/she feels so empowered that the adventure of life can be embraced in joyful expectation, could be regarded as having gained a good deal from his/her therapy. A perceptible refashioning during cognitive-behavioural therapy of the self-destructive thoughts (meticulously recorded in the first of the typical run of six sessions) into self-constructive thoughts (recorded with equal meticulousness in the last of the typical run sessions) appears to be a patently obvious substantiation of that form of therapy. If an 'eclectic' style is utilized, then the therapist may combine methods of assessing the productiveness of the therapy, or select one which he/she considers the most appropriate.

However, what if in the psychoanalytical/dynamic example, all that is happening is that spurious connections are being made between two unconnected events? In the second example, what if the client is ending therapy because she/he is dissatisfied with its quality but doesn't want to upset the kindly therapist? With reference to the third example, might it not be that contrasting 'destructive' and 'constructive' thought-processes (and linking these with emotions and behaviours) is so supremely complicated as to be a delusional venture for short-term therapy? In the last example, doesn't the lack of any semblance of a theory–practice system, and the vagaries of personal choice, fuel such a high level of subjectivity that it might be more appropriate to abandon assessing effectiveness rigorously altogether or to stick with the inanely subjective (and all too common) question 'How was it for you?'?

Consider the following scenario: our client, Heather, following her earlier brief encounter with the Jungian therapist, heads towards her first brush with a humanist mind-healer; after two telephone calls and a lot of fiddling with dates and times, Heather has a date in her diary on a day suitable more for the therapist than for her; Heather, distraught by her troubles, has been told by friends that she really does 'need help' (beyond that which Len appears to be capable of giving); regardless of her unrelenting cynicism about therapy, and the dent made in her iron mask of pride because the opinion of her friends is that she needs it, Heather has gone ahead and picked a professional helper from an advertisement in the telephone book (business pages); but, as with the previous Jungian therapy, she does not know the intricate practices of this therapy. Heather has had many intrusive medical investigations, but her fear of psychological surgery is excruciating particularly as she does not want any therapeutic incision to again touch the extraordinarily sensitive region of the relationship with her father. Heather, in her social role of 'client', doesn't know what to expect; she doesn't know if it will make her eventually feel worse or better, or whether she will have to feel worse before she feels better. Heather feels that already the control she tries to exercise over herself and over others is slipping away; being so mentally vulnerable raises her heightened fear to utter dread; but once in the room with the therapist her egotistical superciliousness metamorphoses into edgy submissiveness.

So should Heather at this stage be provided with an account of the debates concerning efficacy? As the rapport germinates, and possibly informal or formal contractual arrangements are discussed and qualifications divulged, might it not be also apposite to point out that the therapy about to be used is underscored by faith or science, and that, if science, then it is also fallible?

Apart from such an elaboration on the evidence (or lack of it) soaking up all of the content for perhaps six sessions, Heather is no fit state of mind to take on board anything other than the apparent convictions of the therapist. She is starting to panic and wants to run away, as she does with most other situations she find threatening, from the impending emotional trauma of revealing and attempting to deal with her troubles. If not 'flight', then Heather may 'fight', and turn hostile towards the therapist. A third option for Heather is to become 'flaccid', requesting the therapist to 'just get on with it'.

Judging whether or not therapy does what it is supposed to do is enormously problematic for anyone, whether client, therapist, or independent researcher. An initial difficulty is that it depends on which one of the escalating number of therapies is being assessed. However, testing the soundness of therapy frequently involves comparing individual therapies (for example, solution-focused with psychodynamic), or one therapy either against or alongside psycho-tropic medication. Next is the problem of choosing the method of judgement. Should it be intuition and experience or science that is called upon to verify a therapy? Although there are still diehard believers in personal insights from case studies as a means of justification (see for example, Charles 2004), the rules of science have encroached on the therapeutic enterprise. Science is used increasingly by both outsiders (perhaps science to attack the value of therapy), *and* by insiders (to help raise the prestige of their field or defend it from other paradigms of psychological intervention such as psychopharmacology). But, science itself, as a way of understanding the world, can be called into question.

There has always been a division within the therapeutic enterprise (from Freud onwards) between those who wish to legitimize what they do by taking shelter under the authority of scientific objectivity versus those who indulge in a faith in therapy. However, the legitimacy of the latter in a 'scientized' world (that is, one in which science is considered the best or the only valid way of understanding physical and social concerns, and 'evidence-based practice' is *de rigueur* throughout public policy) cannot be easily sustained. But the former also has a 'legitimation crisis'.[2] That is, while faith in therapy easily collapses under the discriminating consideration of the sceptic, a good deal of sceptical ammunition has been amassed to undermine (if not demolish) the credibility of science.

In this chapter, therefore, the nature of science is first discussed, and then the 'scientization' of therapy. Next, the proposition from the sociology of scientific knowledge that science is founded on a fallacy is discussed, and whether or not without scientific legitimacy, and despite the deficiencies of science, therapy is no more than snake oil.

Science

Lewis Wolpert, Professor of Biology, University College, London, believes in science (Wolpert 2005). Richard Dawkins, Professor of the Public Understanding of Science at Oxford University (Dawkins 2006), Steven Pinker, Johnstone Family Professor of Psychology at Harvard University (2003), and Ben Goldacre (2008), British-trained medical practitioner and journalist, believe fervently in science. They are science purists. That is, they regard science to be not only the pre-eminent 'body of knowledge' (epistemology) for understanding the natural and the social world, but the only way to understand those worlds. Moreover, they are science evangelists. What they believe is that scientific rules and results should be disseminated vigorously throughout society, and they attack what they view are the myths about, abuses of, and threats to scientific thought. For example, they assail postmodernism (a belief that anything can be believed) and nihilism (a belief in nothing); they consider the use of scientific discoveries to wage warfare as immoral; and view the expansion of religion as not only absurd intellectually, but a downright danger to civilized culture. Such scientific fundamentalists (fundamentalism meaning here purist-evangelism) fear the swamping of society with asinine, primitive, and destructive thinking and practices when what is needed are more analyses and answers from science about such social problems as disease, poverty, and climate change.

However, spreading the glory of science requires a more sophisticated selling technique than just preaching about successes in medicine, physics, genetics, and evolution theory. That has been tried before, and as the preachers of scientific fundamentalism recognize, it has failed. Otherwise the rise in the late twentieth century of alternative medicine, and interest in the paranormal, creationism, intelligent design, and religious fundamentalism (for example, Islamic, Christian, and Hindu), would not have taken place, and science would not have to defend itself. To promote their message what the scientific fundamentalists indulge in is the propagation of 'pop science' in literature (books and articles), and through campaigns (through lectures, conferences, on specialist internet websites, and media appearances). A more evocative strategy is to highlight the beauty and poetry of science. Scientific beauty and poetry, the scientific fundamentalists believe, can be found in all manner of scientific exploration, from uncovering the laws of the universe to grasping the working of bar codes on packaged supermarket foods.

Fits, stops and starts

Science may be beautiful and poetic but how it came about and what it is isn't straightforward (Lindberg 1992). That is, science did not and does not develop in a unilinear and progressive manner by single or groups of scientists having 'eureka' moments whose ideas are universally accepted and who are given public acclaim for their efforts. Science has arisen in fits, stops, and, starts, and continues to stutter along, inter-dispersed with reversals as well as forward leaps. Moreover, some of the most impressive scientific discoveries are a consequence of serendipity, many prestigious scientists really can be regarded as 'mad' in the sense that their discoveries may rock conventional wisdom, and a variety of new age and old age religions continue to vie with science in the twenty-first century for explanatory dominance (Gribbin 2003).

However, there is some semblance of established history to and understanding of science. The ancient Greeks are mainly responsible for setting in place embryonic scientific ideas that were to become modern Western science (Lindberg 1992). Building on the ideas of previous civilizations (for example, Babylonian and Egyptian), Greek science covered medicine, astronomy, cosmology, geometry, mathematics, electricity, magnetism, human biology, zoology, geography, and music. The ancient Romans contributed engineering and technology and further medical knowledge to the science laid down by the Greeks. Both the Greeks and the Romans, however, invented and maintained non-scientific beliefs such as mythology and 'the gods' throughout the rule of their empires (Lindberg 1992).

After the fall of the Roman Empire and the subsequent Dark Ages and Middle Ages in Europe, the science originated by the Greeks did not disappear altogether. Moreover, elsewhere in the world (for example, the Islamic Middle East, India, and China), scientific ideas continued to evolve. But superstition and theology either prevailed as explanatory modes or caused those with a scientific bent to keep a low profile for fear of being demonized.

However, as early as the fifteenth century, science was re-surfacing in Europe. Nicolaus Copernicus (1473–1543), a Polish mathematician and astronomer calculated the positions of the planets and pronounced that the earth revolved around the sun. Italian physicist and astronomer Galilei Galileo (1564–1642) calculated that objects with unlike mass will fall at the same rate, and designed an effective telescope. The European

Enlightenment philosophical movements, beginning in the seventeenth century but much more prominent in the eighteenth century, heralded in both political liberalism and rational (scientific) ideas. This was the Age of Reason. Religious beliefs were challenged, and individual equality and liberty were regarded as basic human rights. For example, the writer and philosopher Voltaire (1694–1778: his real name was François-Marie Arouet) campaigned against injustice, intolerance and bigotry, and for science. René Descartes (1596–1650), apart from rather unhelpfully declaring that the mind was separated from the body (given that this is considered to be misleading by most contemporary Western and non-Western thinkers), was arguably the founder of modern philosophy and mathematics.

Positivist leap

A great forward leap in what is considered to be the platform of modern science was achieved by Sir Isaac Newton (1642–1727). Newton, a British mathematician and physicist, discovered the laws of gravitational force, calculus, optics, and motion. In doing so he firmly implanted into scientific philosophy the 'deductive' method – testing hypotheses, observing the results from these tests, and those hypotheses which are confirmed consistently can lead to universal (scientific) laws. Aided by one of the founders of sociology, French philosopher Auguste Comte (1798–1857), a version of science (that is, 'positivism') that can be tracked from the Greeks through to Newton, has been adopted by most of today's Western-inspired scientific community.

Gerard Delanty (1997) has catalogued the core tenets of positivistic science:

1 Scienticism – only scientific knowledge is credible.
2 Empiricism – we only know what can be observed, and the experiment is the basis of scientific observation (through which 'cause' and 'effect' relationships can be established).
3 All knowledge is susceptible to the techniques of natural science.
4 There is a reality which can be studied, and science stands ('objectively' and 'value-free') outside of this reality.
5 Internally coherent and universal laws exist which cross over bodies of knowledge.

So, for the positivist, society, the mind, *and* therapy can be studied in the same (scientific) way as physics, chemistry and mathematics. For the positivist scientist, mathematical formulae and the laws of physics and chemistry can provide predictions about how a car will run, when the sun will burn out, or when water will boil. The implication is that scientific research into therapy can predict that the repetition of affirmative thoughts will breed happiness, being nice and listening intently will empower clients to take charge of their lives, and exposing conflicts in the unconscious will improve mental health.

Scientific medicine

Science has a long association with (Western) medicine, and serves as a model for the direction that therapy may be heading in. The professional status of medicine is underscored by science, and scientific evidence is expected (by medical professional associations and governments) to be called upon to support all forms of medical interventions. Indeed, government agencies have been assembled to ensure that not only medical practice, but also the practice of the disciplines allied to medicine (for example, nursing, midwifery, physiotherapy, radiography, and audiology) is substantiated by research that meets the rigours of science. However, the evidence called upon by the allied disciplines may not necessarily be unerringly positivistic. Nursing, in particular, has tended to embrace inductive (qualitative) or 'soft' scientific investigation rather than deductive (quantitative) or 'hard' science. A hierarchical ranking of evidence, which in the main has been that derived from 'hard' science on its pinnacle, means that the status of disciplines such as nursing (and to date therapy) is part of the reason that they are not at the same level as medicine.

The linking of medicine to science by organizations representing medical or scientific interests and by the media, is explicit, perpetual, and exultant. Alok Jha, science correspondent of the British newspaper *The Guardian* writes about the potential of medicine to cure many somatic and psychological ailments (specifically, Crohn's disease, diabetes, coronary heart disease, rheumatoid arthritis, and bipolar disorder) following the successful scientific analysis of the human genome:

> Scientists have made a major leap in unravelling the genetic causes of seven common diseases ... The discoveries pave the way for improved treatments and possible cures for the millions of people in the UK who develop the diseases every year.
>
> (Jha 2007)

Founded in 1848, the American Association for the Advancement of Science (AAAS) claims to be the leading voice for scientists globally. Its aim is the advancement of science in society, and since 1880 it has published the prestigious scientific magazine *Science* in order to help achieve that aim. *Science* has a readership of 1 million. Nearly 3,000 articles directly relating to medicine were published in *Science* during the years 1995–2007 (2007, AAAS-*Science*).

Threats to the scientific basis of medicine (and on occasions it is medical practitioners who are the menace) can arouse a considerable defensive reaction and a uniting of forces from the science and medical communities. In 2006, leading scientific institutions in Britain raised their concern that changes to the regulation of homeopathic medicines were likely to harm patient care. The outcry was joined by 600 medical practitioners and medical scientists, some of whom are leaders in their field, who signed a petition against allowing promoters of homeopathy to make claims about its efficacy (BBC News 2006). The pro-science pressure group Sense about Science reported that evidence-based medicine is paramount to public health, and that there is no (hard scientific) evidence that homeopathy contributes to public health (SAS 2006).

Ridicule is also used against those with views and products that are not supported by any science, are anti-science, or are shored up by dodgy scientific claims. Ben Goldacre, author of a regular newspaper column entitled 'Bad Science', wrote good-humouredly, but nevertheless with an undercurrent of witty derision, about his attendance at a famous annual outdoor music event in England:

> I'm dispatching this column to you from the frontline of the healing fields at Glastonbury festival, where I can cheerfully offer aura reading, structural integrative massage, soul therapy in the pyramid healing space, happy footbaths, crystal magick [*sic*], positive thinking yoga and angel therapy. In an angelically charged dome. There are no scientific claims, it's all very cheery, and I honestly don't have a problem with a single thing here . . . Now I wouldn't want you to think that I've gone soft in the head, or that I've been packed into a wicker man by a slowly advancing circle of angry hippies . . . Okay, maybe I feel a bit iffy about premium rate chatline millionaire astrologist Jonathan Cainer who's speaking later on, but right now I am sat outside the Gong Bath tent: 'the most powerful form of holistic resonance known to man'. You lie on a bench – blindfolded – while a man walks around you ceremonially playing two gongs, really quite loudly.
>
> (Goldacre 2007a)

Goldacre's quasi-seduction by hippies was temporary it would seem. His mission to educate the public about medical 'quackery' versus medical science, the 'bullshit' of perpetual motion versus laws of thermodynamics, about the villains in the media and dissenting scientists, and especially the dangers of homeopathy, continues unabated (Goldacre 2007b; 2007c; 2008). Moreover, for Goldacre, scientific medicine is not only important (it demonstrates what can kill or cure), but also elegant and beautiful.

Scientization

The Strasbourg Declaration on Psychotherapy of 1990 defines psychotherapy as an independent *scientific* discipline. But, unlike medicine, only parts of the therapeutic enterprise have a compelling and genuine allegiance to science, and some parts are not just un-scientific but anti-science (especially the 'alternative', constructionist, and postmodern therapies).

Moreover, some of the declared associations of therapy with science can be considered rather dubious. For example, the American Psychoanalytic Association (2007) states on its website that it is an affiliate of the American Association for the Advancement of Science. It has a large caption advertising this affiliation, along with a direct internet link to the website of the American Association for the Advancement of Science. This is an interesting affiliation as it cannot be held that psychoanalysis is scientific without some considerable qualification.

Freudian quackery

Freud was originally a neurologist, and therefore trained scientifically. Paul Broks, senior clinical lecturer at the University of Plymouth, UK, and honorary consultant neuropsychologist, goes as far as suggesting that Freud can be deemed as not only the founder of psychoanalysis but also the science of neuropsychology. For Broks, Freud stimulated a huge amount of curiosity about the nature of human personality, the self, and especially the unconscious, and his ideas remain popular. But Broks concludes that most if not all of Freud's ideas remain within the category of 'abstract notions' rather than scientifically validated realities:

> Freudian language has seeped into common parlance like that of no other writer since Shakespeare. The core ideas of his psychoanalytic theory have become part of the fabric of our culture. Accounting for human behaviour in terms of unconscious thoughts and hidden motivations has become commonplace. We all know about wishful thinking, about denial and defence mechanisms, repression, narcissism, Freudian slips and the anal personality. [But it] ... is not just that so

much of Freudian psychology seems nebulous and fanciful: in certain regards it is patently wrong. His ideas on female sexuality, for example, are rightly derided (penis envy, the inferiority of the clitoral orgasm).

(Broks 2006)

Nor can it be easily proclaimed that psychoanalysis is accepted by the public or academics as having the same prestige as quantum mechanics or astrophysics. Consequently, the American Psychoanalytic Association's identification with a high-status scientific body could be understood as a strategy to massage its own standing and that of (one type of) therapy. Moreover, the American Psychoanalytic Association is a component of the International Psychoanalytical Association (2007). But the International Psychoanalytical Association does not ally itself with any organization that is overtly scientific, and has a very wide research brief (which includes scientific study but also 'scholarly', conceptual, philosophical, historical, and naturalistic investigations).

Pretentious psychology

Psychology, the parental discipline of the therapeutic enterprise, also indulges in status manipulation concerning its association with science. Besides the American Psychological Association, another national agency representing psychology in the USA is the American Psychological Society (established in 1988). However, the American Psychological Society underwent a name change in 2006 and became the Association for Psychological Science (2007). The Association for Psychological Science is a fervent sponsor of science in psychology, with the express mission to promote, protect, and advance science in the teaching of psychology, psychological research, and applied psychology (including therapy). Underscoring the Association for Psychological Science's dedication to science are its journal publications, all which have 'psychological' and 'science' in their titles: *Psychological Science*; *Current Directions in Psychological Science*; *Psychological Science in the Public Interest*; *Perspectives on Psychological Science*.

The practices of therapy have been studied comprehensively. But, again, therapy differs from medicine and (to a lesser degree) psychology as there is not a whole-hearted use of 'hard' scientific methodology in these studies. When therapy calls upon science to analyse or advertise its efficacy it may be in the form of a 'survey' of what clients think of the service they have received. For example, the British agency *Relate* ('*The Relationship People*') displays on its website the results from two studies which have assessed feedback from clients (*Relate* 2007). These studies (McCarthy et al. 1998; McKeown et al. 2002), using self-completed questionnaires, found that clients were mostly very positive. A large majority stated that they were satisfied with the therapy they received from *Relate,* with a smaller majority believing that it had improved their relationship.

Surveys, while they cannot be accused of being 'soft science', are on the 'soft' side of 'hard' science, as are many research procedures emanating from the social sciences (particularly anthropology and sociology). Questions in surveys relating to what therapists say the therapy should do and whether or not it has done it, or how satisfied clients are with their mind-altering adventure, are self-serving and highly subjective. However, 'hard science' techniques (such as controlled trials) have been undertaken in their thousands, and appear to provide similar conclusions to the surveys: therapy works, therapy is cost-effective, and all therapies are about equally effective (Asay and Lambert 1999).

However, the scientific substantiation of concepts and achievements in therapy (and generally within the mental health industry) remains questionable. An assemblage of academic psychologists, inspired by Scott Lilienfeld (Associate Professor of Psychology at Emory University in Atlanta) has embarked on an exposition of beliefs and practices in the mental health field which they regard as unproven or unsafe. This group, however, is accused by other senior psychologists, who either stick to experience and intuition or who are more tolerant of 'soft' science, of being far too zealous in their devotion to hard scientific method (that is, controlled trials and statistical analysis) to verify theories or testing efficacy (Goode 2004). Certainly, this group is zealous. They are the scientific fundamentalists of psychology.

What originally irked founders of scientific fundamentalists James Wood, Teresa Nezworski, Scott Lilienfeld, and Howard Garb, was the use of the Rorschach Test. For them this test (whereby meanings a client extracts from an inkblot are interpreted by the therapist), used tens of millions of times over decades to assess personality and mental disorder, is bogus. For Scott Lilienfeld, Steven Lynn, and Jeffrey Lohr (2004), there needs to be a clear delineation between science and pseudoscience in clinical psychology. The mission of Scott Lilienfeld and William O'Donohue (2008) is to get scientifically authenticated psychology principles (17 of them) to be embraced by mental health practitioners. Scott Lilienfeld, John Ruscio and Steven Lynn then wish to offer prospective clients advice about which types of therapies (and therapists) to trust and which ones to shun.

Therapeutic efficacy

So, which specific therapies does scientific evidence indicate are recommendable? As with many scientific explanations, the answer depends on who is asking the question, why they are asking, and when it was asked.

Research to date suggests that therapy appears to be effective for approximately two in three clients. Hence, for about a third of clients it doesn't work, and self-help programmes may be equally as effective as professional helping (Bates 2006).

The authors of the 2006 edition of *What Works for Whom: A Critical Review of Psychotherapy Research*, Anthony Roth and Peter Fonagy (and their collaborators) are either senior academics or senior practitioners in clinical psychology. This review of psychotherapy is aimed at establishing the scientific 'evidence-base' within the British NHS[3] for psychotherapy and, to a lesser extent, counselling (which they somewhat sniffily infer is less rigorous in its theoretical foundations and practices than psychotherapy). There is an acceptance by the authors that the review is limited by the necessary selection and classification of particular rather than all of the therapies (they calculate there are at least 400), and by the narrow definition of 'evidence' they adopt (favouring controlled trials). Therefore, they caution:

> Reducing evidence to a binary option of supported or not supported is not an adequate representation of the research literature, and the criteria used to judge whether a treatment has evidence of efficacy will always be to some degree arbitrary. Notions of efficacy beg the question of what is considered sufficient evidence, and what degree of change may be regarded as appropriate or significant.
>
> (Roth and Fonagy 2006: 480)

What Roth and Fonagy conclude is that for some therapeutic interventions there is clear evidence of efficacy for particular maladies of the mind. For other therapies, there is either restricted or no evidence that they work. Instances where there is evidence of significant efficacy include:

1 exposure therapy (in vivo) for specific phobias (such as agoraphobia);
2 exposure therapy and cognitive therapy (in combination with exposure) for social phobia;
3 cognitive-behavioural therapy and applied relaxation for generalized anxiety disorder;
4 cognitive-behavioural approaches and Interpersonal psychotherapy for major depression

5   exposure and response prevention for obsessional-compulsive disorder;
6   cognitive-behavioural approaches and eye movement desensitization and reprocessing for post-traumatic shock disorder;
7   family intervention programs for schizophrenia (alongside anti-psychotic medication);
8   dialectical behaviour therapy and psychodynamic psychotherapy for borderline personality disorder.

Undoubtedly, the above list will alter as data amasses to the support efficacy of other therapies or found to underline the ineffectiveness of others, and so the scientization of the therapeutic enterprise will grow.

But Richard House (2003) has pointed out that those who are unhappy with the therapy they have received may not report their dissatisfaction because they might blame themselves for it not working. Furthermore, House questions the meaning of 'success' in therapy. For example, does it imply that the client has become more happy or just less miserable? But what then is 'happiness' and 'misery', and how much more of one or less than of the other can be equated with 'success'? The placebo or snake oil effect of having faith in what both Thomas Szasz (1978) and William Epstein (2006) have described as the 'religion of therapy' may be what is effective, but then this will only be as usual as either not doing anything or talking to a friend.

Therapeutic alliance

However, David Smail (1999) records that if there is any scientific consensus at all about the success of therapy it is that the personal qualities of the therapist count a great deal rather than the technique employed. This implies, says Smail, that untrained people could be as effective as qualified therapists as long as they have personal qualities that suit the needs of the client.

Roth and Fonagy acknowledge that the 'therapeutic alliance' has to be considered when judging the efficacy of therapies. That is, the relationship between therapist and client may undercut or complement the functioning of any therapy.

Furthermore, Roth and Fonagy accept that there is anecdotal and empirical data about the experience and intuition of the therapist supporting the supposition that the relationship between therapist and client is crucial. If the relationship is not conducive to the needs of the client, then no matter how sophisticated and relevant the technical and philosophical elements of the therapy, they are unlikely to meet those needs. For Heather, 'getting on' with her therapist is paramount. It wouldn't make a difference what regular or fanciful therapy style is used, Heather's habit of jumping to judgements about the worth of people means that if the therapist doesn't give the 'right impression' straight away, then she may either ditch therapy or keep changing therapists until she finds one with whom she can 'get on'.

But, argue Roth and Fonagy, the evidence for the importance of the therapeutic relationship is insubstantial and inconsistent, and that separating out the variable of the therapeutic alliance from the therapeutic content and processes, is exceedingly complicated.

Notwithstanding the clarifications about what therapy works for which type of psychological distress and the impact of the therapeutic alliance, Roth and Fonagy's review of the evidence is sympathetic to the notion that therapy is a worthwhile endeavour. However, there is a far more incisive attack that can be thrown at such an inference: to conjure science as the only genus of knowledge that can (eventually) explain everything cannot be justified.

Fallacy

Science has come under sustained assault from various quarters. Much of the criticism considers its procedures, knowledge, and lust for omnipotence as deceptive if not deceitful. The whole edifice of science, therefore, is perceived to be either 'built on sand', and thereby vulnerable to collapse. But even if science is not about to implode under its own contradictions and broken promises, it is wobbling under the sustained barrage of disrespect, digressions, and disinterest. The use of a wobbly epistemology to buttress the enterprise of therapy is surely somewhat risky.

Give or take a few historical deviations into witchcraft, religion and mythology, and the present-day drift by 'New Agers' back into paganism and the preposterous, science has had thousands of years to get its message across. That is, ever since Ancient Greek civilization, science has either been lingering in the background, awaiting an opportunity to burst forward and knock out its competitors (principally religiosity or mysticism) for epistemological dominance, or has actually attained that dominance.

The European Enlightenment gave rebirth to the scientific ideas of ancient civilizations and birth to a staggering range of innovative ones. Industrialization provided the opportunities to apply these ideas. That was hundreds of years ago. But there is much evidence that the public still do not understand the scientific basis of their world. The journal *Public Understanding of Science* (Einsiedel 2007) registers the persistent misinterpretation of scientific endeavour by, and scientific illiteracy of the public, and examines the dangers to the ideals of the Enlightenment from old and new anti-science movements.

Public ignorance

Science (and technology) form the backdrop to everyday human performance in the twenty-first century. Virtually all the activities that humans engage in, or aspire to, have a technical basis which comes from science: eating (highly technical food and globalized distribution systems; electricity and micro-waves or scientifically engineered gas piping to cook food); travelling (cars; trains; aeroplanes; boats; motorcycles); entertainment (television, DVDs; cinema; sport stadia); cleanliness (showers; washing-machines; dish-washers); or communications (mobile phones; the internet).

But most people could not describe the techno-science that gives them an instant meal with ingredients from a multitude of different countries, allows them to travel to the other side of the world, communicate immediately with others no matter where in the world they are, and brings hot water at the flick of a switch or turn of a knob. Nor are they appreciative of how biotechnology and information technology may rapidly be changing many aspects of human performance (especially values), or of the resultant ethical quagmire (Fuller 1997; 2007a; 2007b). The public's ignorance of and perplexity over science have resonance with medieval perceptions about devilry, the earth being flat, and corn circles (all three of which still have mythical appeal among a minority). Science books written by pre-eminent physicists (Hawking 1995), as well as renowned novelists (Bryson 2003), have become best-sellers. But not as successful as books about wizards and broomstick flying. As if in confirmation of the public's obtuse bewilderment about their scientific world, the internet book retailer Amazon lists *Harry Potter and the Philosopher's Stone* (Rowling 1997) under 'science'.

Scientific fundamentalists, of course, consider the attitude of the public toward their preferred doctrine, as one of educational or intellectual deficit. Sociologists of science tend to project this as an arrogant and ill-informed stance. It is disrespectful of the meanings people give to their lives and other belief systems to which they adhere, and ignores the social processes and structures that shape attitudes and science.

In-house criticism

However, there is 'in-house' criticism of science. That is, some scientists acknowledge that science cannot provide all of the answers to how the universe and its contents work, and that (positivistic) science springs from 'theories' and some of these theories (even the most sanctified) may become disreputable. Other scientists, while retaining a resolute faith in science, disagree with each other over which science has the best answers. Some scientists admit that society affects science.

Hence, scientists (unless fundamentalist in the extreme) are not blind to the shortcomings of science. Moreover, these shortcomings have been recognized by scientists throughout the history of science. Indeed, the theoretical foundation of science was not originally considered a threat but strength. Bertrand Russell (1961) noted that the Greeks did not separate philosophizing from their accounts of natural events. To the Greek scientists, 'thinking' about reality was as important as 'discovering' reality. Scientific knowledge may be concerned with objectivity (concentrating on the production of 'factual' statements about 'real' phenomena), but it is also heavily speculative. All statements of 'fact' are mediated through conjecture. Natural laws (for example, gravity, and the 'big bang') are speculations on the real world. All knowledge (whether scientific or not) succumbs to social processes in its production. It is not, however, inevitable to conclude from this that knowledge is fabricated totally, or that science is as good or bad in terms of an accurate exposé of reality as any other system of ideas.

Moreover, philosophers of scientific method disagree with each other about how to conduct science, and scientists actually conducting science disagree with the philosophers and with each other. There is much controversy within science about whether or not science should proceed 'inductively' (start with the evidence and then look for the theories) or 'deductively' (start with the theories and then look for the evidence), amalgamate induction and deduction, or pick the most appropriate depending on what research question is being asked. Moreover, if deductive, then there are problems of 'verification' (without empirical evidence, a theory is meaningless) and 'falsification' (theories have credibility only if they are capable of being proven to be false). Although generally science proceeds deductively, enormously important subjects in science are to date unverifiable and unfalsifiable (theories about the big bang, superstring theory, and much evolutionary developmental psychology).

Whatever the in-house controversy, scientists in the main consider their knowledge to be progressing. Newtonian physics was replaced by Einstein's, by 'big bang' by 'superstring', superstring by 'M theory'. But these are all advances not retrenchments.

Thomas Kuhn

However, the iconoclastic claims of science historian Thomas Kuhn (1962) continue to have resonance in debates about the credibility of science. Kuhn argued that there are long periods of 'normal science' in which researchers accept the presumptions of their predecessors and contemporaries. During 'normal science' scientists operate within an accepted paradigm of thinking and practices, and for the most part do nothing more than address particular puzzles that were internal to that paradigm. Only those problems are researched, and conclusions sanctioned, that make sense, given the principles of the paradigm. Evidence that springs up during the period of 'normal science' which contradicts those principles or stands completely outside the paradigm is dispensed with through mockery or is contained through the formation of theories that are in tune with the paradigm.

But, suggested Kuhn, at various times in the history of science, the build-up of evidence repudiating the accepted paradigm becomes so great that it starts to disintegrate. This heralds an era of 'revolutionary science', a time of turmoil within the scientific community with much uncertainty and contention about what can be classified as authentic knowledge. At the end of the revolutionary interval, a new paradigm will emerge, and a period of 'normal science' will ensue – until the process starts again. Who knows, homeopathy and hands-on healing *could* have their day in the epistemological sun.

'Epistemological arrogance' is at the heart what Nassim Taleb argues is the delusion of 'normal science' today. Science can only convince itself and try to convince everyone else that the universe and its contents can be understood by keeping its thinking 'inside the box'. The plausibility of 'deductive predictability' is only possible because science has set out its own rules of discovery. This is intellectually fraudulent, however, as the natural and the social world is much more prone to randomness. Things happen far more by chance than science acknowledges, or has the tools to acknowledge. Heather resolving her troubles after ten weeks of humanistic warmth and genuineness may be recorded as a successful outcome for that therapy and that therapist. But she may have resolved them anyway in ten weeks (unlikely), with or without the aid of her sporadic alcohol and chocolate excesses. Or a bout of the persistent tapping of the body advocated by 'thought-field' therapists might have done the trick. Alternatively, if the therapist had an ability to 'think outside the box', (which Heather was able to do from time to time), there might have been a sweeping reconfiguration both to her troubles and their resolutions.

'Normal science' is not in any case an homogenous discipline. As Steve

Fuller (2007b), Professor of Sociology at the University of Warwick, points out, finding common ground between scientific sub-disciplines is problematic. Physicists, chemists, mathematicians, palaeontologists, and geneticists are exploring different – and frequently incompatible – domains. To transfer the rules and predictions of quantum mechanics to the study of fossils or DNA is perhaps in itself a fabricated, and therefore unscientific, process. Steven Rose (1997), Professor of Biology at the Open University, argues that *within* each scientific sub-discipline there are rival explanations of natural phenomena.

Contamination

'Objectivity', the cornerstone of positivistic science, is seriously contaminated by the availability of financial support and by how effectively research conclusions are disseminated and implemented. What is studied, and how it is studied, depend, to a large extent, on funding. Obtaining funds depends on whether or not particular organizations (such as drug companies, government departments, charities, and lotteries) consider their commercial, political, or public and 'humane' interests will be met by the research findings. It is rare to find tobacco companies, breweries, or the arms industry, subsidizing projects that aim to investigate the damage smoking, alcohol, and guns do to health. If they do provide funding for such research, then their motivation may be questioned (perhaps their generosity being a public relations exercise under the banner of 'corporate social responsibility' as opposed to genuine philanthropy), as will the ethics of the researchers for accepting funding from these sources. The results of such research will almost certainly be perceived to be tainted. Fiscal concerns will encourage politicians to be wary of supporting research into, for example, new medical treatments or the plight of the elderly, if this might lead to demands for expensive treatments and increases in the state pension.

Moreover, researchers embarking on areas of interest that either do not require funding or attract financial sponsorship from organizations that are more liberal in what their money is used for, are from the outset engaged in the subjective selection of their topic. It is the individual researcher's 'interest' that drives him/her. This interest may not necessarily be disconnected from the priorities of global society (whatever they might be, and whoever might identify them). However, it may be very idiosyncratic with little obvious substantial benefit to anyone other than that researcher.

Beyond commercial manipulations of medical science, science generally is stage-managed by politicians. Politicians (and medical insurance companies) are much more amenable to funding research into, for example, relatively low-cost short-term therapies than high-cost and long-term, and allow the cheap therapies to be offered in health services. Heather is more likely to be offered by her general practitioner, if offered anything at all (other than a five-minute placatory chat and some anti-misery medication), cognitive-behavioural therapy or solution-focused therapy than she is psychoanalytical/dynamic therapy (Leader 2007).

The neo-conservative administration of US President George Bush was accused of manipulating science to support its political ideology. Thousands of scientists (including 20 Nobel Prize winners) signed a petition against the distortions engineered, they claimed, by the US government concerning a wide range of health and environmental policies (Buncombe 2004). Similar accusations of political misuse of scientific evidence were made about the British Government of Tony Blair. The British Parliamentary Select Committee on Science and Technology (2006) reported that government ministers had been selling some of their policies to media and public by falsely claiming that they were upheld by scientific evidence. Politicians, recommended the committee, should be honest and declare when they are advocating policies because of 'conviction' and when there was 'evidence'.

More subtle commercial manipulation can occur, for example, in the paying for the research papers to be 'ghost-written' in a manner that hides the negative effects of a business corporation's products or promotes its new products. Prestigious medical academics and practitioners are then asked by pharmaceutical companies to add their names to these papers so that they are taken by the wider medical community to be authentic (Fugh-Berman 2005).

'Peer review' is hallowed by the scientific community. For example, *Sense about Science* (2008), the science lobby group, considers peer review as the most viable way of disseminating research findings and thereby contributing to authentic knowledge. Researchers, wishing to publish their findings, submit articles to journals with scientific prominence (for example, *Science* or *Nature*), and/or with an ethos of 'evidence-based' practice (for example, the *Lancet* or *Therapy Today*). The process of reviewing these articles is projected as objective and authoritative. Typically, the reviewers (who may or may not be part of the editorial team of the journal) recommend a submitted research paper for acceptance, amendment, or rejection. However, the editorial teams of academic journals and the reviewer, appointed in the opinion of the editor(s) for their 'expertise' or as a consequence of personal associations, are themselves part of a scientific establishment that has preconceived interests and values with regard to what is and what isn't genuine scholarship. Such appraisal, rather than being authoritative and objective, is pooling subjectivity. Furthermore, the existence of a hierarchy of scientific journals which is employed by academic and research authorities, puts immense pressure on researchers to publish only in those journals that are at or near the top of this hierarchy. The criteria for publication in prestigious journals are, by definition, highly rigorous, but as a consequence of such rigour, also exceptionally narrow. Therefore, the subject and method of inquiry (positivistic science), and the medium of disclosure (peer review in scientific/evidence-based journals), are pre-given. Under these conditions it is exceptional for a dissenting, imaginative, 'out-of-the-box', author to be given the opportunity to be published.

Smail (2002) comments that the scientific core of psychology (and, by association, therapy) is bogus. Reference to other peer-reviewed articles to support a researcher's own conclusions relies on the belief that knowledge is cumulative and incontestable. This is, for Smail, absurd because there is no delving into the arguments and nuances surrounding the previous published work. Smail (2006) also criticizes the 'mechanized' methods of science which exclude obvious unscientific (but nevertheless relevant) factors. Scientific enquiry (and an extremely narrow and tyrannical variety at that) has become the most important way of earning income to the detriment of what universities were originally designed for: thinking and emancipation.

Out-house criticism

The sociology of science (or what is becoming known as 'social epistemology: Fuller 2007b; Goldman 1999), recruiting ideas from Kuhn and Foucault, has led the 'out-house' criticism of scientific knowledge. At the core of this critique is the constructionist proposition that knowledge of any sort, whether emerging from a traditional source (for example, magic, witchcraft), co-existing lore (such as alchemy, metaphysics, celestial prophecies, psychoanalysis, paranormality, and religion), or science, is bound by historical circumstances and cultural norms.

That is, as Michel Foucault argued (1969), what we think of as unalterable 'facts' or unchallengeable 'truths' (at various times this might be 'God exists', 'doctors are gods', or 'cognitive-behavioural therapy is a god-like panacea'), are *always* contingent on the cultural and historical contexts in which they were manufactured. The belief in an omnipotent Christian god could not have been upheld without the institutions of Catholicism and Anglicanism, and the power-broking that has occurred with various state authorities over two millennia. The medical profession gained its professional dominance and clinical autonomy in the nineteenth century by winning inter-occupational battles for governance over human life and death.

Postmodernists are the fundamentalists of constructionist thought. Scientific medicine, quantum mechanics, superstring/M theory, Buddhism, Judaism, Christianity, Islamism, socialism, capitalism, holism, or humanism, are all social constructions. Each one is only 'true' or 'factual' if we care to view it that way, but there is in reality (and of course there is no reality but endless possible realities) no real truth or real fact. Something only appears to be truth or a fact if it has been awarded that status by those with an authority to do so. But with any issue, there may be competing authorities.

Frequently, there is contrary scientific evidence about health. Take multivitamins as an example. Scientific evidence from, for example, the Harvard Center for Cancer Prevention, Harvard School of Public Health[4] (2007), using a summary of data accumulated until 2005, states that multivitamins taken daily can protect against a number of chronic diseases, including some cancers (there are also studies which indicate that multivitamins slow down HIV and Alzheimer's disease). But other scientific studies suggest that multivitamins might be very dangerous to the health of men because taking them correlates with cancer of the prostate (BBC 2007). Such disagreement gives sustenance to postmodern views on multivitamins: first, they are a 'commodity' rather than a necessity for survival; and second, contradictions in the evidence demonstrate that science is flaky (as is every other 'knowledge').

Girl Guides

Postmodern life is made up of a multitude of possible truths in a world where everything has been fashioned into a commodity, factual basis to human performance, only lifestyle choices. Motherhood for Heather is not 'natural' fact, and the unnaturalness of her experience of being pregnant and giving birth has been a worry to her for years. She loves children and is excellent with children, but admits she has no instinctive 'female' drive to nurture. She tends to assume traditional masculine characteristics with the Girl Guides troop she runs weekly, and when looking after her friends' children as well as her own. Moreover, her first husband Saint, father of her two children, is much more motherly than Heather. Although Heather does not identify herself as a postmodernist (or a radical feminist), her attitude to and feeling about being a mother illustrate the point that the seemingly most basic truths (mothers have an inborn love for their children) and 'fact' (mothers are feminine) are socially constructed norms from an earlier epoch and may have outlived their shelf-life. What has worried Heather, however, is not that she does rate motherhood or want to be motherly, but how she is perceived by others – particularly other mothers. When she left her first husband and children, she was plagued by a concern that she would be regarded as an appalling woman. Her idea of motherhood did differ markedly from those around her, and she did receive abusive comments from other mothers when she collected her children from school and attended school festivities.

But, a postmodernist (or existential) therapist would propose to Heather that whatever role she chooses is no better or worse than any other. This is the freedom our postmodern life offers to us.

Summary

Therapy has moved in the direction of scientizing its practices. However, what scientists project arrogantly as evidence should not be taken at face value. Science is implanted in myriad of social contexts, and therefore, what is cast as 'real' without uncoupling these contexts is suspect.

Neither a scientific fundamentalist nor a fundamental constructionist, Simon Blackburn (2006), Professor of Philosophy at Cambridge University, argues that the search by scientists for truth and facts should be respected, but we should be sceptical about them ever achieving this goal.

Brian Goodwin (1997), a Professor of Biology (at the British Open University) takes the view, an unusual one for a scientist, that while there is a real world to be studied, any knowledge of this world will only be an interpretation rather than fully truthful or factual. Subjective opinions and social processes inevitably interfere with the search for facts and truths. Goodwin's (2007) solution is the formation of a new culturally-sensitive and holistic science, which understands these interferences.

The sociological theory of realism acknowledges that scientific knowledge is fallible (Bhaskar 1998). Realism accepts that what can be known about a 'real' entity is mired in social constructions. But the realization that science is fallible should not lead automatically to the conclusion that nothing can be explained through science and make us adopt the methodological anarchism of Paul Feyerabend (1975) that substitute epistemologies will do any better, or that blind faith is good enough. Scientific methods can offer insights into what we understand our existence to be, but human intuition, introspection and experience also contribute 'knowledge', including that which relates to therapy.

Perhaps a realist conclusion about the credibility of science is to amend

Winston Churchill's famous 1947 dictum about democracy thus: science is the worst way of looking at the world except for all the others that have so far been tried (Morrall 2008). Perhaps a realist conclusion about therapy is that its arrogance is not yet justified but may be eventually, and that it may offer Heather some insight into her protective shield of arrogance.

CHAPTER 4

Selfish

> Individual
>
> Reflexive
>
> Sexualized

Therapy is exceedingly 'selfish'. That is, the therapy enterprise is compulsively obsessed with the 'self'. At the heart of enterprise of therapy is the self. Its values and practices are imbued with numerous connotations of the self. Without the self, therapy has no *raison d'être*. If the self did not already exist, then therapists would have to invent it.

Each therapy session revolves around 'selves'. Ideally, the therapist, through training, experience, and supervision, is highly self-aware and projects his/her professionalized 'self' with the aim of being therapeutically effective. The client (or clients if couple, family, or group, therapy) presents his/her 'self', perhaps initially in a disguised or protected form, for either the known or unknown purpose of it being discovered, accepted, reformulated, or 'actualized'.

Heather is also selfish. But Heather's self is also muddled. She is in a constant state of discomfort with her self, unable to rest easy with her own psychological make-up. Her self is not just muddled, but is heavily disguised and defended. Consequently, Heather does not really know herself *and* fears knowing her self.

To be fair to Heather, all clients (and therapists) are selfish in the broader meaning of the term I am using here. My meaning encapsulates not only the egocentric and incessant orientation towards 'me', but also the prevailing and compelling movement globally towards the individual as the locus of human activity and input.

But what is the self, and what does sociology have to say about whatever it is? In this chapter, the very idea that there is a 'self' is considered not as a natural or a God-given, integral, and inevitable constituent of humanity, but as an outcome of certain social processes. These processes are, it is argued, responsible for either accentuating or manufacturing individualism in society at the expense of collective patterns of human activity.

Two specific sociological versions (reflexive and sexualized) of the self are then explored. These accounts detail the social impetuses that are moulding the self in today's globalizing society. Heather, as expected, makes regular appearances, as her 'self' (whatever that is).

Individual

The self and therapy go hand in hand. Most of Freud's intellectual and therapeutic work focused on the psyche, and in doing so located much of human distress within the individual (specifically, on one or more specific regions of his/her mind: the id, ego, and superego). Psychoanalysis is in essence 'analysis of the self' (with the analyst usually analysing his/her own self before embarking on the analysis of their client's self). Freud did not ignore the impact of society on psychological distress (Bocock 1977). However, undoubtedly Freud is the most prodigious promulgator of selfishness within contemporary therapy *and* a significant force in the furtherance of individualism in Western society at large. Notwithstanding his realization that society had a great deal of influence on how the mind developed normally and abnormally (especially in the formation of the superego), his contribution to comprehending human performance,[1] and also that of many of his successors, concerns the intrinsic and intricate mental activity. Anna Freud (1936), his youngest daughter, was particularly instrumental in the promotion of the self with her work on child psychological development, and the ego and its defence mechanisms.

Sinister

But the self uncovered by Freud is a very sinister self, especially within its unconscious arena. Although mollified by protective apparatus that attempt to instil psychological calm, the self is perpetually strained. For Freud, the unconscious is riddled with dark desires, usually connected to violence and sexuality, but also life-sustaining facets. On the one hand, it is molested by incestuous commands, destructive forces, and procreative drives. On the other hand, it is inspired by benevolence and creativity.

Freudian considerations of the self provide a clue as to why Heather has troubles. It could be that she is so unsure about her self, and behaves so erratically, because of unresolved pressures in her deep and hidden self.

Freud and post-Freudians were party to the prolific social changes which occurred throughout the twentieth century. Frank Tallis (2005), in his account of the history and unhealthiness of romantic love (for Tallis, 'being in love' should be classified as a mental illness), notes that references to the self as a substantive psychological entity can be traced back to the seventeenth century. Robert Burton's methodical study of depression contains a detailed dissection of the self (Burton [1621] 2001).

But, latter-day rampant consumerism, invention of highly sophisticated medical technology for inspecting and fixing internal bodily functioning, and mapping of the human genome, have encircled the individual and furthered the significance of the self. Humanity in Western culture has become anatomized, and the self has triumphed above considerations of group identity (such as the family and community). The self is now hallowed, indulged, eroticized, improved, asserted, disciplined, and mourned.

The Victorians were interested in the self. In 1859, the same year as Charles Darwin published *Origin of Species*, Samuel Smiles published the best-selling (and still in print) *Self Help: With Illustrations Character, Conduct and Perseverance*. However, my (non-scientific) investigation of self-help literature on sale in a local bookshop, in August 2007, found over 400 different titles – and that did not account for self-help material contained in the health, religion, social science, mind and body, and sex shelves. Titles included: *The Complete Idiot's Guide to Verbal Self-Defense* by Lillian Glass; *What to Say When You Talk to Your Self* by Shad Helmstetter; *Self Esteem Bible* by Gael Lindenfield; *Self Matters* by Phillip McGraw; *The Successful Self* by Dorothy Rowe; and the promisingly ironic *The Last Self-Help Book You'll Ever Need': Repress Your Anger, Think Negatively, Be a Good Blamer, and Throttle Your Inner Child* by Paul Pearson. Using the term 'Self-Help' to search the internet store Amazon produced nearly 40,000 book titles (books, CDs, and DVDs) and the internet search engine came up with over 41,000,000.

Moreover, the march of the self continues with the conquest of global society in its sight. Collective human arrangements for living such as communism and socialism (albeit as bastardized versions: the former Union of Soviet Socialist Republics, the People's Republic of China, and the Socialist Republic of Vietnam) have been or are being swept aside, are economically debilitated (for example, the Democratic People's Republic of [North] Korea), or only serve as a cultural irritant to individualized nations (the Republic of Cuba's relationship with the USA, where individualism is revered, being the obvious example).

Good

However, it was Carl Rogers who was to place the self at the heart of the therapy and humanity (Purkey and Schmidt 1995). He regarded the self as the core of what is to be a person. Both therapist and client for Rogers not only had to have a self, but it had to be a very special self: genuine, honest, unconditionally respectful, warm, empathic, and capable of actualization. This type of self, for Rogers, was what therapy, and every other type of human interaction, should be based on. Humanistic, client-centred therapy and its therapeutic offshoots, together with the majority of other styles of therapy including psychodynamic therapy (but not necessarily psychoanalysis), use this idealized self as a fundamental starting point for their practices. To be effective, the Rogerian therapist has first to realize that she/he has to have this idealized self (through a programme of self-awareness), and then use it purposefully during verbal and non-verbal communications with the client. The Rogerian therapist also must believe that every client (and every other human) has a similar self. If these admirable qualities of the client's self are not apparent, then the therapist has the task of exposing them. An appropriate physical environment in which to conduct therapy, and an array of communication skills, will enable the emergence of the client's 'good' self. For Rogers, when enough individuals return to, and trust, their 'good' self (through therapy if necessary), social ills such as criminality, avarice, aggression, and suspicion would be wiped away: good selves make good societies.

From a Rogerian perspective, Heather is doing the best she can. She, like all humans, is fundamentally a good person, who is struggling to make sense of her self, her family and others associated with her, and her society. Humanist therapy offers a route for the subdued and submerged goodness of Heather to ripen and displace the auto-injurious and flinty aspects of her self.

Determined

But if the self is me, what is the me that I am? Am I sinister or good? Moreover, how did I get to be this self? That is, is the 'self' the consequence of genes which have been designed through evolution, and determine much of human performance including what we become as individuals? Or can individuals circumvent their biological inheritance and construct their own version of a self (for example, through therapy), selecting what and who they wish to be and able to change when they wish to do so?

Biological determinism has its equivalent in sociology. Extreme structuralism implies that what individuals experience as their 'self' is the product of the social environment. Consciousness, freedom of expression, and ability to think, are induced by forces in society beyond an individual's control (arising from, for example: gender and ethnic role expectations; and economic and political ideologies and policies). From the structuralist viewpoint, transnational corporations are intoxicating and indoctrinating the individual, refashioning him/her into a mass consumer. Moreover, electronic communication is becoming as common as face-to-face contact. There are now trillions of communicative impulses zooming around cyberspace.

Electronic communication and media technologies are moulding 'me' into a 'cyberself' with shifting virtual identity (or identities) intermingling with or extending the 'real' self, or spawning a 'second self' (Strate et al. 2002; Turkle 2005). Humans do not transmit messages to each other when in close proximity in the same way as they do when typing and sending a message to a loved one, friend, colleague, or therapist. Moreover, whether or not electronic communication is occurring in 'real time' or with a considerable time delay may disrupt the intended meaning and the projected imagery of the selves of both sender and recipient. However, Schultz (2001) argues that electronic communication is not necessarily qualitatively different from face-to-face communication. That is, it is not inevitable that talking with an embodied person means that there is better understanding taking place than with a disembodied person. For example, the social surroundings of a discussion between a therapist and a client may be detrimentally affected by preconceived views about the other's identity (for example, ethnic group, gender, or age). But communication via email, internet, or the telephone (mobile and landline) while losing non-verbal clues and cues, has the advantage of camouflaging the social status of the participants. It therefore becomes more egalitarian and more in-depth, suggests Schultz. However, the therapeutic enterprise has yet to assimilate and decipher the nature of electronic communication and the nature of the therapist's and client's self when therapy is conducted within cyberspace.

For scientific fundamentalists such as Lewis Wolpert (2005), the social environment (and that must include cyberspace) does affect human performance, but its effect is limited by genetic inheritance. The fact that human language is universal demonstrates the biological heritage of human performance. The content of human speech is inspired by culture (it is unlikely that evolution would pass on conversational topics such as the latest television soap opera plot or intrigue about the personal assignations of popular football players). But the genetic endowment of neurological circuits, developed in embryo, enable humans to talk in the first place. Whether biological or social, or a mixture of the two, if human performance is pre-ordained to a large if not total extent, then the therapeutic enterprise has the serious problem of authenticity. The enterprise of therapy bases much of its business on the notion that humans are unique as individuals, and that change for the individual is possible. But, if individuals are prisoners of their biology and/or society, then therapy cannot help to ascertain, mould, or liberate the self. It is perhaps a tribute to the marketing strategies of the therapeutic enterprise, given that these are hardly delivered coherently, that therapy is becoming more and more saleable and not a product past its sell-by date.

Neuro, cognitive, and evolutionary sciences are producing intriguing insights into the self which are altering our perceptions of the self. The brain has been shown to have sufficient plasticity to allow alterations in both physical and mental functioning, and the mind is being mapped as a thinking and feeling computer, with malleable software but an inherited hard drive (Buss 2003; Thagard 2005; Doidge 2007).

Escaping

Eminent sociologists Stan Cohen and Laurie Taylor's (2004) thesis is that humans spend much of their time trying to be other than the self society wants them to be. Existence is either so boring, so traumatic, or so constraining, that 'escape attempts' are made constantly. People, faced with increasingly routinized, regulated, commercialized, consumerized, homogenized, monitored, and controlled lives, are in a bind. They, desperate to display their individualism and avoid the reality of their ultimate demise, engage in a range of supposed self-liberating and self-reaffirming activities. These include: recreational sex; romantic encounters and literature; criminality; protests and revolution; music; sport; painting; singing; dancing; yoga; and therapy.

Escape, while possible, in the main is delusional. Much of what is escaped to is eventually enveloped by the exigencies of the economic and political power from which the individual was trying to escape. For example, self-expressive hobbies may well be operated by large commercial companies, adventure travelling is a major part of the tourist industry, and ecological and voluntary work has proliferated beyond personal altruism to corporate 'social responsibility' and 'volunteerism'.

Regulated

But Nikolas Rose (2007), Professor of Sociology at Goldsmiths College, University of London, sets out to debunk the self altogether. For Rose, borrowing imaginatively from the work of Michel Foucault, claims the individual is not a real entity but a cultural artefact. Historically, Rose suggests, the individual has not had a significant and stable cultural meaning until relatively recently. It is Western society, over many centuries, which has steadily created a discrete entity, an encased singular human with his/her own physical and psychological composition, and biography.

Specifically, the growth of capitalism needed individualism to furnish its continued expansion. Commodity fetishism and consumerism are conditions in the self that are paramount to global capitalism. Latterly, this process of individualization has gone further by amplifying the importance of a particular portion of the individual that has become known as the self. The globalization of (Western) culture has transported individualism to nearly every part of the world.

Rose (1990) also argues that along with a culturally recognized individual and the self has come enhanced freedoms and rights but also regulation. The regulation of the individual is occurring in two directions: (1) increased surveillance of individual conduct; and (2) increased self-control. Both directions, states Rose, lead to 'governance at a distance'. Rather than governments directly intervening in the lives of people to ensure adherence to the requirements of the new world order (global capitalism), individuals are encouraged to comply because they know they are being watched and they are also internalizing a mantra of self-responsibility. Those who do not comply and perform as 'good citizens', are demonized (witness the moral panic in Britain over paedophiles, mad murderers, criminal recidivists, and binge drinkers).

Moreover, Rose (1985) points out that it could only be in an individualized culture that the discipline of psychology could emerge. Psychology, broadly the study of the mind of the individual, has produced a discourse about the self and by doing so has reinforced the self as a reality. Thus psychology is the servant of the economically powerful – those who benefit directly from the manufacture of a culture that emphasizes the individual.

Psychology is, argues Rose, a 'constructed domain'. Rose uses the term 'psychologization' to describe how psychology has infused society with 'truths' about the mind. Psychology has, just as medicine did (which also was only able to ascend the occupational hierarchy through individualism) when embarking on the medicalization of society, enlisted science to support its spread of influence. But psychology's scientific pretentiousness is therefore a contrivance aimed at defending its complicity in the rampant individualization of global culture.

Rose is fully aware that the discourse of psychology is disunited, having, as it does, competing perspectives on the self. But he reasons that it is psychology's diversity that allows a thorough colonization of the psyche. That is, by not having a fixed target for its critics and competitors to aim at, it is hard to kill off or supersede. Diversity also means that it can infiltrate further, proliferate more effectively, its individualized conceptualization of humanity.

The discourses of psychology, along with psychiatry, have entered prisons, courtrooms, schools, the workplace, hospitals, retailing, the media, and entertainment. In its expert and its 'pop' forms, it is called upon to give intelligible explanations for the normal and abnormal working of the mind, judgements about sanity, insanity, innocence and guilt, methods to change behaviour, business management, punishment techniques, treatments, epistemological endorsement of therapy, and rationales for the plethora of self-help programmes.

Together with medicine, psychology guides and manipulates the life of the individual, and what he/she considers as his/her 'self', to a considerable extent. However, unlike medicine, psychology's success, posits Rose, is due to its simplification of many matters relating to the psyche (especially by means of popularized literature and television programmes) as well as diversity. While impenetrability (through, for example, using a mystifying language) helped medicine to achieve dominance over the health of the individual, penetrability has allowed psychology to 'govern the soul' and 'shape the private self' (Rose 1990).

Foucault (1981) has already observed how the self has become 'confessed' in contemporary society. We want to know about our self and to tell others about our self (Foucault is referring particularly to our sexual self). Therapy has become the most patent avenue for self-revealing, and psychology affords therapy the conceptual language which can be adopted to deliver the confession.

Heather has bared bits of her self to her various therapists (and much more to Len, her barefoot therapist). Naked, her private self becomes exposed to public inspection, probing, comprehension, and renovation.

Heather being Heather, however, is resistant to psychological naturism and therapeutic fondling. She rebels against what Foucault regards as the disciplining of the self, and takes her undisciplined self out of therapy.

Reflexive

George Herbert Mead (1934) was one of the first sociologists to combine the self (and its mind) with society. His variation of sociological interactionism, known as symbolic interactionism, has been very influential in sociology. Erving Goffman furthered symbolic interactionism, taking it through a number of developmental stages (phenomenology and dramaturgy). He was then able to produce his seminal works on how the self is 'performed' in everyday life (Goffman 1959), stigma and 'spoiled identities', and the institutionalizing and normalizing effects of 'total institutions' such as the asylum (Goffman 1961). Symbolic interactionism is still called upon to provide research theory for empirical studies which examine social phenomena microscopically, and a number of current theoretical positions that attempt to link human performance at the level of the individual to that of society (although Mead himself did not fully achieve this difficult sociological feat). The linking of individuals with society is referred to as 'reflexivity', although this term has alternative meanings (for example, in research it infers the purposeful involvement of the researcher in the research process; in medicine, it means an autonomic bodily response, in popular usage, reflexive tends to be used as a synonym for being reflective).

Conversation of gestures

Mead theorized that the self was understandable not as an organic entity, but as the result of a process involving a constant 'conversation of gestures'. Gestured conversations (verbal and non-verbal communication) between humans, especially those who have significant relationships with each other (family members, teachers, lovers, partners, and peers) give relentless clues about the individual's self-identity. These clues, particularly if the same ones are repeated, become internalized and form the way in which that person comes to view his/her self. This impression, first provided *by* others, is then offered *to* others. If the projected self is reinforced through further positive verbal and non-verbal feedback, then this variation of the self is stored within the organic substance of the mind, and is used again. If the feedback is such that this self becomes challenged, then the content and style of the self are reviewed by its proprietor. If consistently negative, and the negative is supplied by numerous significant others, the individual will amend his/her self. In its modified state, the self is tested for further encouraging or discouraging feedback. The process of presentation, review, and modification continues (for life).

As a sociologist, however, Mead had to consider the self more than simply the consequence of interpersonal signalling and intrapersonal dialogue. The signals and dialogue, for Mead, have to have a social origin. What the self becomes is an interactive and dynamic importation *of* influences from others and society (what Mead calls 'social attitudes'), and an exporter of influences *to* others and society.

Therefore, Mead also questions the reality of the self. He certainly does not believe that the self has an existence 'for itself', but is a part of the multifarious organizations and processes that form a society. The individual's self represents not itself but society. There is no self, mind, personality, or intelligence without spoken and unspoken signals, and these signals belong to, and are tendered, by society.

Me and I

However, the individual does experience his/her self as real, owned by him/her unless he/she is an infant, psychotic, senile, or drug abuser. The individual's self is usually also perceived by others as real, and is related to in that way. To explain the apparent discrepancy between a socially owned self and the personally owned self, Mead refers to the 'I' and 'me' split. The 'me' is the self that humans present to the outside world (the self as-known), whereas the 'I' is what individuals present to their inner world (the known-self). That is, what an individual regards, on introspective examination, as his/her real identity (character, beliefs, feelings, and thoughts) is what he/she thinks of as the 'I'. What an individual shows to, and what is observed by others, is the 'me'.

So, for Mead, the self is in conversation with both others and with itself (the 'I' and the 'me'). That means that there are incessant adaptations and adjustments occurring constantly within the self, between the self and others, and between a population of selves and their society. This may give the impression that individuals and societies are sitting on shifting sands of interaction. However, for most of the time the self and society are functionally stable. Generally, unless in times of psychological or social collapse, or major personal or social change is deliberately instigated, the movements that are taking place are imperceptible, and core segments of the self and society remain relatively untouched. When change for both individuals and society takes place, in the main it does so slowly as the means of change can only emerge from the internal and external conversations. The means to think and interrelate are embedded in these conversations, which themselves are embedded in the society within which they are taking place. The human self, for Mead, is both the product and producer of society.

Not for turning

Can Mead's symbolic interactionism give insight into how Heather sees her self? The fundamental bits of Heather's self that might be responsible for her troubles would be very difficult to transform, if they needed transforming in the first place. Moreover, they could only change if therapy directly and powerfully intervened, and she participated willingly and vigorously, to dislocate the patterns well established through four decades of conversational input. Heather is much more likely to engage in a 'conversation of gestures' that echoes a declaration made by Margaret Thatcher (British Prime Minister from 1979–1990, and first woman to hold that post), when being taunted by her political (male) enemies within her own party to ditch her radical monetarist economic policies: 'Turn if you like, the lady's not for turning'. Thatcher persisted to the bitter end of her political career, which ended only when she was unceremoniously 'asked' to resign by her own ministers, to assert that her policies were right. This earned her the reputation of being a political visionary, committed, resolute, unnervingly truthful, *and* stubborn, domineering, adversarial, and gratuitously uncaring (Yergin and Stanislaw 1998). Thatcher, while head of the Conservative Party (which, as its name implies, conventionally has stood for the retention of or return to 'traditional' values), and leader of a profoundly conformist nation, considered herself a 'rebel leader'.

Heather has much in common with Thatcher. She, like Thatcher, can be considered: a creative thinker (although her well-toned humour and intelligence are lethal weapons and are sometimes employed with caustic effect, they do lead her to make many extraordinarily shrewd and witty observations); dedicated (she is, by and large, faithful to her partners, and despite her avowed lack of maternal instinct, she adores her children, and is a devoted and skilled teacher of children and highly regarded in her role as leader of a Girl Guide troop); determined (if she gets the bit between her teeth about an issue will persist until she achieves her goal, or until she exhausts herself trying); and candid (thereby presenting as 'an open book', if one with a few pages stuck together which are thus unreadable). However, as with Thatcher, Heather can be regarded in a harsher light: obdurate (unwilling to readjust her opinion, to admit despite incontrovertible evidence that she is mistaken about an issue or she misunderstood the intentions of others); overbearing (her vigorous assertiveness can give the impression of imperiousness); adversarial (while heroically confronting those who, for example, make racist, sexist, or homophobic remarks, she can also 'explode' with her family, friends, and lovers); and hard-hearted (rarely and mostly inadvertently, Heather appears numb to the feelings of others).

But if Mead is correct about the formation of the self being the product and producer of society, how could Thatcher have become such a 'conservative radical'? How does Heather make such ingenious and hilarious observations on life, as well as avoid substantial negative feedback? Neither Thatcher nor Heather should have the ability to so dramatically and innovatively 'think outside of the box' if the human self is so tightly colluding with society and is so susceptible to signals from others. Mead's model of the relationship between the self and society is one of reciprocation, and has the organization of society and of human thoughts changing only gradually. Put simply, the human mind cannot think *beyond* society because it *is* society.

Indeed, Mead states quite clearly that no one person can alter the whole of society. He provides the example of how a politician with a project (always a worry to the civil servant overseers of the status quo), will have formulated his[2] ideas from 'conversations' received from various segments of society and from his colleagues. That is, his 'me' has been communicating with (and in this instance, actually listening to) others. The politician will have digested these messages and added his/her own elements and interpretations. That is, his 'I' has had its input, and along with the 'me', his self has made up its mind. For Mead, this is an example of what he describes as a 'great co-operative community process'.

Well, Margaret Thatcher during her reign as Prime Minister was most certainly uncooperative (to large swathes of society, and to many members of her own political party), made far-reaching social changes (dismantling large segments of the welfare state), and managing to swing public support to fight a war (over tiny territories thousands of miles from Britain). It is yet to be seen whether or not Heather will do the equivalent at her workplace or in the Girl Guide movement.

Moreover, Mead's model means that therapists who regard a thorough renovation of their clients' performance as a goal have a somewhat forlorn task. In the face of a deluge of gestures from the rest of society (or at least the client's significant others), fortifying existing performance or otherwise pulling in only a moderately different direction, Oedipal analysis, client-centred kindliness, or cognitive-behavioural 'mind-bending', are doomed to failure.

Structuration

Anthony Giddens (1984; 1991) takes up the theme of 'voluntarism' versus 'determinism'. He has tried to bridge the gap between those who believe that humans act voluntary, have free choice, and self-consciousness (this includes most psychologists and therapists, and some sociologists), and those who argue that human behaviour is largely or completely dictated by the social circumstances and dominant ideologies in which they exist (the belief of structural sociologists and unreconstructed social workers). Giddens synthesizes the two extremes of voluntarism and determinism, claiming that humans do have choice in what they think, do and say, but this is constrained by social factors (as well as biological dictates).

Individuals, for Giddens, belong to a society that has pre-given structures. Rules, laws, roles, and relationships make up this structure. Formal and informal norms and mores indicate what is acceptable and what is unacceptable human performance. Humans, however, think for themselves, interpret and provide 'meaning' for their own performances and those of others. They are reflexive, constantly examining, and aware of major public issues (such as warfare, abortion, sexuality, violence, alcohol and drug abuse) as well as their mundane own everyday concerns. The term Giddens uses for this reflexive process is 'structuration': individuals and social structure are interrelated; human performance generates the content and form of society's structures, and society's social structures generate the content and form of human performance.

So, the construction of the self for Giddens is one that is an amalgamation of personal choice and social prescription. Take the analogy of going for a meal in a (French) restaurant, which has an *à la carte* rather than *table d'hôte* menu. The diners can select their own combination of foods rather than having the selection limited to exactly what the chef decides they should have. Through making their choices, the diners are very likely to influence what will be made available for future menus. Of course in both instances the chef has the upper hand in deciding what foods to have in the restaurant. Moreover, a choice can only be made from the ingredients available in the markets (although today these extend well beyond the local). Similarly, freedom for the individual and the shape and range of the self are contiguous on society (and biology). 'Thinking outside of the box' is a misleading concept: the individual can escape the boundaries of the box (which he/she has already helped to build through the process of reflexivity), but will find he/she is then sitting in a bigger box.

Alterations to and expansion of sexuality, the rise of consumer lobby groups, vegetarianism, terrorism, alternative lifestyles, and therapy, have all come about through self and society transactions. A few individuals may have given the impetus for changes in sexuality, and increases in punter power, non-meat eating, violent politics, and holistic holidaying. The relevant social institutions will have in consequence responded, and in the cases cited encouraged more individuals to follow suit. The reverse is also possible. It could have been the social institutions that initiated the first action, and a number of individuals then reacted. Social institutions with the biggest impact on individual performance include the agencies of government, global corporations, and the mass media. For David Gauntlett (2002), the way the modern mass media operates is a prime example of the reflexivity, as described by Giddens. Television soap opera storylines and advertisements portraying families as comprised of marital disharmony, sexual infidelity, and an embarrassment of consumer goods, together with news and documentary programmes that reinforce this impression, become appropriated by individuals.

Reflexivity, suggests Giddens, occurs both externally (between the self and society), and externally. Self-identity is thus 'made' and is continuously 'remade' through reflections about what society is indicating human performance should be *and* through the individual considering how his/her own 'biographical narratives' fit into the demands of society. Biographical narratives comprise, for Giddens, the story that individuals invoke about their self: the type of person they are, their personal histories, and futures they want for themselves. Giddens, like Tallis, blames the eighteenth-century upsurge of romantic love. Being in love necessitates assembling a story about our self, that of our lover, and then a combined story about the joining of these two selves. The conjoint story then has both a past and a future, and becomes the backdrop force for the account of the lives of the people concerned (for as long as the 'sickness', as Tallis views romantic love, lasts).

People attempt to maintain a core self-identity made up of their own biographical narratives. However, the extremities of their self-identity, and sometimes the core, are alterable through reflexivity. Giddens accepts that the self is a modern cultural phenomenon, especially in its highly reflective state. The obsession with self-reflection (which therapy exacerbates), along with the malevolent effects of modern mass media, creates an uneasiness in the core self. Giddens refers to wobbliness in the core self as 'ontological insecurity'. Heather is certainly wobbly.

Giddens observes that 'living in the world of late modernity' endows the self with various tensions. The self is in danger of fragmenting because it has to deal with so much reflexivity and is aware of having to be a different self, to a greater or lesser extent, in a host of different circumstances because the world has opened up and become visible. Furthermore, in this open and visible world, which has become so through travel for the masses and mass media, the self has uncountable choices available. Choosing lifestyles for the self intensifies ontological insecurity.

If Giddens is correct, then what seem to be tensions owned by Heather's self are not hers as such, but result from 'living in the world of late modernity'. She is part of this world, and therefore has to accept a certain amount of responsibility for contributing to its problems, but her self can hardly be blamed for the process of reflexivity from which fragmentation and insecurity exude.

Giddens, despite his distaste for unadulterated postmodernist sociological precepts (but an obvious taste for unadulterated pre-modern political adornments: in 2004 he became Lord Giddens), has a postmodern bent. He refers to the questions everyone has to repeatedly ask themselves in late modernity such as, 'What to do? How to act? Who to be?'. These questions are indicative of postmodernist reasoning about the potential for individuals to build any self-identity or multiple self-identities because the conventions for human performance are either absent, multifarious, or nonexistent.

Notwithstanding Giddens's deviation, the modernist envisions that the self is knowable. Science, for the modernist, can find the answers to 'What to do? How to act? Who to be?' by scanning the brain, mapping the genome, theorizing about evolution, and conducting experiments on cognition. A lot of information is already known about the self, and eventually everything will be known about the self, postulates the modernist. The self is liable to be conceived as a bundle of neuro-transmitting cells and specialist genes with a prolonged heritage to their function.

Saturated pastiche

There is, however, observes Kenneth Gergen (1992), a new understanding of the self that defies the modernist conceptualization. The world has become over-populated, and there is no sign as yet of the birth-rate slowing. This means that human interaction has also increased appreciably. Global society has become 'saturated' with selves. We are bombarded with human contact. There is little private space in which Gergen's postmodern self can find solitude.

Things have got even worse since Gergen first wrote about saturation. Electronic communication has added considerably to the lack of private space, with the virtual world (particularly, mobile telephones, television, and the internet) encroaching on a society teeming with interpersonal exchange, either wanted or unsolicited. Furthermore, the intensity and variety of human relationships have also increased. Never before in the history of the species have humans had such a throng of virtual and tangible friends, lovers, acquaintances, associates, colleagues, teachers, health workers, family members, and people attending to their consumer requirements, as they do in the twenty-first century.

For Gergen, social saturation has resulted in the self being defined by relationships. What the self is depends on the nature of the social interaction in which the individual indulges. The myriad of communications coming from this interaction reduces if not dispels autonomy. The self becomes what others want it to be, and has little if any room for manoeuvre, let alone reflexivity.

The self, hence, becomes a pastiche, a hotchpotch of characteristics which it takes from, or has thrust upon it by, the medley of relationships occupying its social space. Moreover, the sheer number of relationships determines that most are superficial, which implies that the self becomes a conglomeration of shallow meanings and responses. Such a self is not really free to formulate its identity. Gergen suggests the self will eventually cease to exist in its own right. By perpetually constructing and reconstructing itself, the self will become wholly dependent on others for survival. If all selves are going through interdependent immersion at the same time, then presumably humanity becomes a rippling pool of amorphous identities – an unmanageable hyper-reflexivity.

Perhaps Heather's troubled self, therefore, is not just saturated from attempting to surf the tsunami of social change, but drowning.

Sexualized

Either through reflexivity or saturation, society and the self are drenched in sexuality.

> An ever expanding range of commodities is sold by invoking sexual imagery, while sexual desirability is increasingly presented as a leisure commodity to be acquired and utilized, whether in relation to self of others. We live, in short, in a sexualized world.
>
> (Hawkes 1996: 1)

The drenching of Western society in sex has been happening for centuries (Foucault 1985). However, it reached a revolutionary period commencing in the 1960s due to the liberalization of attitudes generally and the liberation of sexuality from procreation with the invention of chemical contraception specifically. Towards the end of the twentieth century sexuality began a second revolution as a consequence of new technologies and globalized trade. Moreover, assisted by the profession of medicine and the therapeutic enterprise, this second sexual revolution, is spreading across global society (Foucault 1985; Hawkes 1996, 1999; Hart and Wellings 2002). As sexual practices transform, sexuality has entered a moral vacuum.

Eroticized body parts of women and men are used to sell cars, tyres, boats, computers, clothes, toothpaste, alcohol, and cigarettes. The display and trading of 'adult' imagery and services permeate the internet, popular magazines, and the pay-per-view television channels of hotel chains. Tens of millions of vibrators and other sex toys are sold each year globally, mainly supplied by China from possibly as many as one hundred thousand factories (Rohen 2006). Sales of sex products and potions within China are worth around US$20 billion, and in the USA pornography is a US$10 billion industry (Rohen 2006). 'Cyber-dating' and 'cyber-mating' (contacting and flirting with potential sexual partners, and maintaining sexual relationships, via the internet) are becoming normalized. Email 'spam' offers to upgrade sexual potency, a bigger penis, or a rejuvenated vagina. Mainstream literature and cinema encompass a flourishing 'erotic' genre, and most books, films, DVDs, and television programmes have either murder or sex as part of their plots or both. Not just the middle-aged but the elderly are expected to retain sexual viability. Hardcore sexual wares are sold openly in many European, North American, and Australasian cities, and prostitution has become legalized or tolerated, Viagra and its competitors allow sexual engagement to be available 'on-demand' and lengthy.

Repression and oppression

Overall, the effect on *Western* society of this sexual flood has been the shifting of sexuality from procreation (having sex to have babies) to recreation (enjoying the pleasures of sex for their own sake). But, there is a paramount sexual paradox in *global* society. In theocratic, fundamentalist, and totalitarian countries, as well as areas of the West that are influenced by right-wing religious groups, there has been a marked increase in sexual repression and oppression. Moreover, for George Frankl (1979/2005), the sexual liberations of twentieth-century Western society have become distorted by, and subjugated to, a market-orientated society. Through the internet, globalized sales of eroticized literature and entertainment, the ease of cross-cultural travel, and sex tourism, not only has the world become 'sexed up', but sexuality is metamorphosing, and new maladies, deviances, exploitations, and sexualities have emerged.

There is the horror of HIV/AIDS, and an increase in the incidence of old and novel sexually transmitted diseases spreading across the world that is barely being contained by health personnel (who are not helped by the dangerously absurd beliefs of some senior politicians in countries most affected by these diseases). The enslaving and trafficking of women and children for prostitution are now a foremost concern of international police agencies such as Europol and Interpol. The sexualization of childhood (for example, by fashion industries), underage/teenage pregnancy, and paedophilia, have become major moral problems.

Gender-bending metro-sexual hermaphrodites

From the soaking of society in sex, a multitude of sexualities has been ejaculated: heterosexuality; bisexuality; homosexuality/lesbianism; transsexuality, and inter-sexuality. There has also been a sanctification of sexual abstinence, and even virginity is making a comeback.

While the debate continues between sociologists, evolutionary psychologists, and geneticists, about how much 'gender' (male or female performance) is determined by 'nature' or 'nurture', sexuality is crossing the boundaries of gender-specific styles. That is, particular sexual patterns are not necessarily confined to one particular gender (and how many genders, and masculinities and femininities, there are is also contentious). Humans may be turning into gender-bending, metro-sexual hermaphrodites. Moreover, whatever the gender performance, sexual practice, or genital equipment chosen, can be discarded for another set at will. Our sexuality hence is not just altering but constantly flexible.

Romans, Greeks, Peruvians, and Victorians

This is not to infer that Western society invented sexuality. What the Romans (and Greeks) did for us, apart from inventing central heating, is to leave a whole host of sexual tracts and habits to be in subsequent cultures either regularized or demonized. The ancient Peruvians also, as is demonstrated by the collection of erotic ceramics housed in the Museo Larco (2007) in Lima, knew far more about sexuality than is strictly necessary for the act of human reproduction.

Liza Picard's (2006) investigation of life in London during the years 1840–1870 explains that the famed prudish Victorian society had an underbelly of salacious sexuality. London, with its much smaller geographical area and population than today, had 3,325 brothels and nearly 10,000 prostitutes, according to police records for the year 1841. Pornographic literature was on sale everywhere (except railway stations). The clitoris, having been found and its purpose appreciated by Greeks and the Romans was seemingly lost during the Middle Ages. However, it was rediscovered by renowned medical practitioner George Drysdale. In his book *The Elements of Social Science* (1861), he covers in great detail the anatomy, physiology and pathology of male and female reproduction, venereal disease, and prostitution, along with discussions on poverty, Malthusian laws of population, and the political economy of the working class. On the clitoris, Drysdale states:

> In the anterior part of the vulva is a small erectile organ, analogous in form and structure to a diminutive penis, differing however in not being perforated by a canal. It is called the *clitoris*, and is highly sensitive like the glans penis. It is probably the chief organ of sexual enjoyment [for women].
>
> (Drysdale 1861: 64)

Drysdale is against sexual abstinence, arguing that it is natural and healthy to exercise every organ of the body. But he is not for masturbation, referring to the 'baleful effects' of solitary indulgence. For Drysdale, masturbation wrecks one's health. He cites cases of adolescent boys spending much of their day 'exciting their seminal emissions' up to twenty times. Physical and mental exhaustion, emaciation, morbid shyness, and possibly idiocy and insanity, may be the result of extravagant autopleasuring.

Male *and* female masturbation is now considered not only normal but healthy. Moreover, alongside the multiplication and fluidity of sexual identity there has been widening of the parameters on what is acceptable or at least no longer taboo: cunnilingus and fellatio; 'swinging'; heterosexual and homosexual anal sex; sadomasochism (bondage, whipping, and spanking, either separately, sequentially, or simultaneously). This is borne out by the proliferation of sex literature in bookshops, subjects discussed on prime-time television/radio programmes, and apparatus and lotions readily available in main-street sex shops and chemists/pharmacies to ease the passage of pleasure and pain while indulging in these practices.

While predominantly heterosexual, Heather has had a number of long-term intimate relationships with women both as a teenager and in later life, and does not rule out more in the future. She hasn't yet decided whether or not she is lesbian, straight, or bisexual, which is somewhat unsettling for her self and presumably the selves of her partners. But whether with male or female partners, Heather needs to either dominate or to be dominant, to be either completely in control, or totally out of control. There is no mediation between restraint and abandonment. Ironically, Heather is able to enjoy abandonment *through* restraint. Unsure of the confines of her self, she found being bound to be comforting as well as arousing.

Handcuffs

However, using fetters to unfetter sexuality is becoming common. An 'outdoor pursuits' shop in the city where I live (York, England), sells steel handcuffs (with keys). Let me be very clear. By 'outdoor pursuits' I am referring to such items as tents, sleeping bags, and sweat-releasing T-shirts, not equipment for orgies *al fresco*. Accepting that embarrassment is a small price to pay for the sake of science, I have conducted 'trials' (uncontrolled but somewhat random) to ascertain why handcuffs are retailed alongside emergency whistles and long-life socks. That is, I questioned different shop assistants on three separate and unannounced occasions in 2007–2008. Further research needs to be conducted, but the limited data from this study indicate that handcuffs are indeed contributing to the sexualization of this relatively small and conservative city (they are selling 'very well' according to my informants), along with the input from the three hard-core and two soft-core sex shops, and a surfeit of 'massage parlours' and 'escort agencies'. Perhaps it's a fitting cultural development, given that York has a renowned Roman heritage.

Moreover, sex drugs such as Viagra are doing more than merely improve performance. They are re-fashioning human sexuality. Popping-a-pill for immediate sexual engagement replaces the need for prolonged eroticized courtship, romantic dinners, and late-night coffee. We can be perpetually prepared for sex, and in doing so it moves mating further and further from procreation, and perhaps beyond recreation towards habituation. Humans no longer need to have babies or even enjoyment when having sex. Sex may soon become similar to the mind-numbing compulsiveness of other popular cultural 'advances' such as television-goggling and shop-shuffling.

Surveillance and control

But, although sexuality in its many guises was known to, and enjoyed by, the Romans, Greeks, and Peruvians, this does not imply that it is a pre-given or natural 'fact' of human life. For Michel Foucault (1985), sexuality (which is to be distinguished from physiological mating) is yet another social construction. Foucault argues that Western society's fixation with sexuality has been manifested through the medical and the therapeutic 'confession'. Sexual preference, performance, and perversions are revealed to the doctor and/or therapist, and in doing so sexuality becomes central to 'self-identity'. This, for Foucault, allows for the further surveillance and control of sexuality.

Indeed, therapy is obsessed with sex. Modern therapy began with psychoanalysis, and as Foucault observes, psychoanalysis always had a zealous concern with sexual symbolism. Moreover, for Foucault, psychoanalysis has assisted in the construction of Western sexuality. Thomas Lacquer, apart from writing about the intriguing subject of the 'cultural history of masturbation' (2003), has also accounted for Freud's legacy for Western sexuality (1990). Freud, posits Lacquer, highlighted the importance of sexuality to the human condition; viewed sexuality and gender as psychological (and social) processes rather than a pre-given natural phenomena; gave credence to children's experiences of their sexuality; indicated that there were powerful unconscious drives to human sexuality, some of which continue to challenge Western social mores.

Sex in therapy

Psychoanalyst Wilhelm Reich's (1989) depiction of the orgasm to prevent and cure mental disorder (through the release of 'orgone energy') is particularly stimulating. His prolific work on sexual climax between the 1930s and 1950s rubbed the custodians of social mores up the wrong way as much as Freud had done earlier in that century. Bizarrely, however, Reich received a two-year custodial sentence in the USA for contempt of court relating to his experiments with 'cloud-busting' rather than 'climax-discharging'. He died in prison.

Gestalt therapy at one time was fanatical about sexual freedom, viewing it as the cornerstone for the full social and political liberation of the individual. Gestalt guru Fritz Pearls assisted in the liberation of some of his clients by having sex with them (Feltham 2007). The intimacy of the humanistic client-centred relationship inevitably is tinged with sexual chemistry (Russell 1993). The conditions of empathy, unconditional positive regard, and congruence, as Carl Rogers (1951), founder of humanist (client-centred) therapy records, can lead to the surfacing of sexuality and has to be guarded against.

Furthermore, the uncovering of childhood sexual abuse is *de rigueur* during therapy. Relationship issues, which may have sexual problems as their cause or as their effect, are abundant in therapy. Problems concerning sexual arousal and performance can come the way of therapy rather than medicine. Therapists have taken on new psychological distresses associated with the global electronic age, such as addiction to internet pornography.

Specialist therapy training and literature dedicated to sexuality is proliferating. For example, attachment-based psychoanalysis for people with issues concerning their passion, longings and fantasies (White and Schwartz 2007); psychodynamic therapy for those with sexual difficulties (Daines 2000); lesbians, gays, bisexuals, and transgender people with 'issues' (Neal 2000); and variety of psychoanalytic perspectives on sexuality (Harding 2001); and sex and the internet (Cooper 2002).

One of the more detailed books on what the therapist needs to know about sex has been written by consultant psychologist and psychosexual specialist Glyn Hudson-Allez (2005). Hudson-Allez covers gender, sex, and sexuality including: genitalia; arousal and loss of arousal; erectile and ejaculatory difficulties; vaginismus and dyspareunia; cross-dressing and transsexuality; sexual addiction; and fetishism.

Relate (2006) on its home webpage advertises its services thus:

Relate, the relationship people – We're here to help you find the answers. Relate offers advice, relationship counselling, *sex therapy*, workshops, mediation, consultations and support face-to-face, by phone and through this website. Here you can find your nearest Relate, book on a course, buy books and consult our experts online. [emphasis added]

It also has a large picture in the centre of the same webpage of a couple under the heading 'Sex Problems'. Below the picture is the following caption:

An active sex life is an enjoyable and healthy part of a relationship. Find out how Relate can help you.

A further boxed caption entitled 'Email a Counsellor' suggests that the reader may wish to email 'one of our counsellors with any concerns or questions about your relationship or sex life'.

Although there have been infamous movements in therapy which have advocated sexual contact between therapist and client, it is generally considered to be absolutely taboo. For example, the American Psychological Association (2008) has since 1989 railed against therapists indulging in sex with their clients. It states that objectivity and trust are destroyed when sex occurs between therapist and client, and is in no doubt that it is misuse of the therapist's powerful position to engage in sex (or to fall in love). But, this very much depends on how sexuality is defined. The American Psychological Association defines 'sexual contact' thus:

> Sexual contact includes a wide range of behaviors besides intercourse, and these behaviors aim to arouse sexual feelings. They range from suggestive verbal remarks, to erotic hugging [non-erotic hugging is allowed] and kissing, to manual or oral genital contact.
> (American Psychological Association 2008; original 1989)

But, according sex enters the therapeutic relationship legitimately as well as illegitimately. That is, sex in therapy can be detrimental or remedial. For David Mann (1997), the therapeutic relationship *is* an erotic relationship. Using the psychoanalytic concepts of transference and countertransference to underpin his argument, Mann reasons that the erotic feelings and fantasies experienced by both clients and therapists are inevitable. Moreover, eroticism can be utilized positively in therapy. Sexuality is integral to the human condition, and therefore to ignore is to repress an integral segment of the client's self and that of the therapist. What Mann is not suggesting is that every therapy session should involve rampant sexual congress, but that sexual histories, feelings, fantasies, metaphor, and imagery should be appreciated and incorporated into the therapeutic relationship.

However, Heath and Len *did* have a full sexual relationship during their five years of knowing each other. What had started as a friendship, moved on quickly to be an informal therapist–client relationship. But the friendship had already begun to be sexualized within a few weeks, at Heather's instigation, of their first meeting. What's worse in terms of crossing the ethical precincts of (formal) therapy, they fell in love.

Summary

René Descartes, philosopher and mathematician, proclaimed that scepticism was essential for intellectual and scientific inquiry. But he was not sceptical about the existence of his self. For him, if he was capable of thinking (and he must have been so capable to have thought about scepticism), then *de facto* he existed. Descartes' ([1637] 2007) renowned Latin axiom, *cogito, ergo sum* ('I think, therefore I am') rests on the notion that human existence depends upon a subjective appreciation of the self.

However, there are alternative comprehensions of the self. The objective perception of the self is gaining considerable momentum. Scientists are seeking answers (perhaps *one* answer) to everything, including 'What is the self?'. Sociologists are never likely to manage to agree on *one* theory for anything, let alone concur over a theory of everything, but all agree that factors external to individual thought are important.

Sociological perspectives on the self include: the self has become targeted and amplified in an expanding capitalist global society that requires hyper-consumerism for it to persist as an economic system; humans are endeavouring incessantly to flee the selves they really are because the reality of existence for many in global society remains as 'solitary, poor, short, nasty, and brutish' as is was in Thomas Hobbes's seventeenth-century England (Hobbes [1651] 1998); both the self and society are mutable and mutual, each affecting each the other; the self is socially constructed, it does not have essential existence; postmodern society and cyberspace have liberated the self, but the self, while free, is also frightened; the self is a jumbled accumulation of contributions from the countless hordes with whom each self has unavoidable acquaintance in the overcrowded world in which today we find our selves; aided by the obsessions of the therapeutic enterprise, a significant outcome from consumerist, saturated, and reflexive society, is a sexualized self.

It is no wonder, therefore, that Heather has egocentric but muddled and wobbly self, and that she had sex with her (barefoot) therapist.

But, although therapy is overflowing with sexuality, Heather's formal therapy sessions (accepting that she only had a handful, and that she had more than one therapist), made little headway in revealing, let alone comprehending, her non-conformist erotic and gender inclinations. No headway at all appears to have been made within the therapeutic enterprise to comprehend or reveal the social context of sex and the psyche since Freud.

CHAPTER 5

Abusive

Power
Control
Sickness

Therapy is abusive. While empowerment is claimed to be at the heart of therapy (McLeod 2003), the therapeutic enterprise, institutionally, intellectually, and interpersonally, has a disempowering effect on its clientele.

Therapy is engorged with power. Power permeates all areas of therapy. It pervades therapeutic relationships, stalking the crevices of the thoughts, emotions, and behaviours of the participants. Power is embedded in the theories of therapy, with assumptions of influence oozing from each concept. The institutions of therapy attempt to wield power in society, over their membership, and, by default, over those who wish to have no part in their power games.

Such virulent power is inevitably open to abuse. However, the abuse I am referring to here is not the blatant form of misconduct such as sexual exploitation, financial irregularity, or academic pretentiousness. Those abuses occur in most social and business enterprises, much is known about them, and the moral debate about them is in the main settled. For example, sweatshop factories and 'modern slavery', enforced prostitution, witch-doctoring and snake oil selling, and copyright and patent infringements, have been exposed and understood for what they are (intellectually bogus and ethically odious). What is far more insidious are not the surmised, and in some instances the well-recognized abuses perpetrated by the enterprise of therapy, but the unidentified or unadmitted perpetrations.

Specifically, the ability of an individual to change his/her personal circumstances through therapy is dictated, limited, or moulded by 'social power' which is external to, and beyond the influence, of the client (as well as by the power of biology). Potent social factors include the influence of close family and friends, the physical environment, and the actions of governments and global corporation. To give the client the impression that he/she has the power to overcome these socially generated obstacles is as abusive as shackling a child to years of hard labour in a clothing factory or a young woman to a domestic setting, buying the services of a captive migrant sex-worker, or manufacturing and selling mock medication to the desperately ill.

Furthermore, another significant abuse by the enterprise of therapy is the (heavily disguised) role it plays as an agency of social control. It does this in two ways: (1) by closing the social space between the twin controlling measures in post-liberal society, self-regulation (individuals monitoring and controlling their own behaviour) and demonization (the targeting and punishing of certain groups which do not self-regulate); and (2) through its undeclared contribution to the 'sick role' (the way in which society controls the deviance of sickness).

So, the therapeutic enterprise absorbs power, sucking it up voraciously and dribbling it out discretely, hiding its dynamic encompassment of power behind a cloak of discursive and practice embellishments. This cloak has the unusual facility, however, of misleading not only the onlooker but also the wearer.

Duplicity also prospered within Heather and Len's affiliation. Theirs' was an abusive relationship.

Power

Susan Jeffers, the self-help guru who wrote *Feel the Fear and Do it Anyway* (the book's advertising blurb states that it has been published in 100 countries and translated into 30 languages), provides a description of individual power:

> I am talking about *power within the self*. This means power over your perceptions of the world, power over how you react to situation in your life, power to do what is necessary for your own self-growth, power to create joy and satisfaction in your life, power to act and power to love. [emphases in the original].
>
> (Jeffers 2007: 32)

For Jeffers, the individual has the power to take control of his/her life. Recognition and implementation of this power, she states, will mean that the individual will never again make a wrong decision or make a mistake, be conned, have low self-esteem, or say no to anything ever again. Reading the book and carrying out the suggestion exercises will result in that person becoming assertive, loving, trusting, satisfied, joyful, and purposeful, with his/her dreams turned into realities. One of the exercises (for women) recommended by Jeffers in order to tap into this internal power is to repeat at least 25 times daily: 'I am powerful, and I am loved; I am powerful and I am loving; I am powerful and I love it'.

Such programmes of empowerment, in various guises, percolate the therapeutic enterprise. Proclamations of the power of the individual to change his or her life, whether chanted or merely assumed, neglect the effects of social power.

Beautiful therapists and clients

An appreciation of the impact of social power on the individual does not negate the existence of personal power. Motivation, wisdom, eloquence, and beauty modulate social power. A shiftless, obtuse, incoherent, and unattractive therapist is likely to be somewhat disempowered by an enthused, astute, erudite, and beautiful client.

Heather is sporadically enthusiastic, habitually astute, effortlessly erudite and indubitably beautiful. Her dealings with formal therapists have been, except for one occasion when Heather could do no more than cry and her therapist no more than 'be with her' (and provide tissues), very much a test of will. That is, Heather, aware of the aura her outward self conveys, looked for a similar 'presence' in a therapist. That didn't happen. The few that Heather met as a client, while not exactly apathetic, stupid, inarticulate, and repulsive, were in her assessment 'not up to the mark'. At her best Heather is instinctively charismatic, and much like the fabled instinct of an animal when it smells fear, she recognized on introduction whether or not a therapist was nervous of her or had the measure of her. All had displayed some degree of apprehension when meeting Heather, and consequently Heather displayed frustration and boredom until at the end of an initial session she could escape never to return.

Len, the barefoot therapist, was 'no oil painting', as Heather was keen to remind him whenever he touched on, no matter how obliquely, innocently, or humorously, anything to do with her sense of dress, weight, or appearance. But despite his artlessness in the realm of female sensitivities, he made more headway with Heather than did her formal therapists. This was largely because he was a strong personality (if not a little too effusive), lucid (perhaps verbose is more accurate), and knowledgeable (although hardly a 'cultured' man, he did, as Heather admitted begrudgingly, 'know stuff'). He could and did use his personal power to challenge Heather. However, Heather in turn used her personal power to evade the challenges, turning interchanges between the two into a struggle for supremacy rather than a collaborative endeavour aimed at resolving her troubles. No matter what the good intentions of Len to assist Heather in resolving the issue of the day, and Heather's lack of malice aforethought, predictably the two would 'lock horns' and grapple with each other psychologically (and, intermittently, physically).

Apart from the personal qualities the participants bring to a therapy session, power therefore will also be mediated by the symbolic interaction between therapist and client. Denis McQuail (2005) has analysed the exploitation of power in interpersonal communication. Monopolizing the conversation can have the effect of gaining control and achieving a desired outcome. Where dominance occurs, and goes unchallenged, the greater the influence. A person can ensure a message is accepted by making it coincide with the beliefs of the other person. The influence of the communicator will also be determined by the content of the message. For example, the influence will be greater if the topic under discussion is an issue with which the other person has no personal experience. Individuals who are regarded as credible and having high social status (as well as physical allure, linguistic and cerebral dexterity, and passion for their subject) will be in a powerful position to impose their opinions.

Powerful status

French and Raven (1959) and Collins and Raven (1969) have formulated a typology of the meeting points of personal power and social power. That is, they divide personal power into a number of categories using criteria derived from statuses ascribed by society:

1   *Expert power*: experts are given a powerful social status for their specialist knowledge; although there has been a demise in deference to experts (within some Western societies), medical practitioners, lawyers, university professors, architects, engineers, and computer scientists, are examples of groups with power through their expertise; the dawn of the 'expert therapist' is yet to rise fully.

2   *Coercive power*: direct physical control, either sanctioned by the state, is exercised over others; coercive power is either sanctioned by the state (police officers and prison wardens), accepted as a cultural norm (parents), or instigated illegitimately (school bullies; kidnappers); coercion may be enacted through psychological interventions such as behaviour-modification 'time-out' (where someone with a mental handicap[1] displaying 'challenging behaviour' may literally be put inside a padded and locked room), or 'holding techniques' for violent outbursts by children or adults in psychiatric institutions; most therapies proclaim an explicit non-coercive stance – their common mantra is 'the client must *want* to change' (however, therapeutic coercion may simply be much more subtle).

3   *Reward power*: emotional or tangible payoffs are given in order to readjust human performance; for example, parents use praise and approval to encourage 'good' behaviour in their children; the therapist's nods or grunts may actively or unintentionally alter the content of the client's story, provide affirmation, or exude disapproval.

4   *Legitimate power*: authorization is granted by the state or other social institutions to employ coercion (law enforcers are trained and tested, and night-club 'bouncers' are licensed), or to exhibit expertise (doctors and lawyers are registered with their professional bodies); the legitimacy of the therapist is inconsistent globally, ranging from being fully authenticated to merely a facsimile of befriending.

5   *Referent power*: acclaim is given for the skills a person may have (sportsmen/women; musicians), his/her social achievements (Jesus, Mohammed, Mother Teresa, Nelson Mandela, Prime Minister Winston Churchill, and President J. F. Kennedy), or his/her academic prowess (Professors Stephen Hawking and Richard Dawkins); added to acclaim is the emulation; acclamation and emulation may be conveyed through sycophantic expressions of deference and veneration; referent power in therapy is offered to the gurus of the enterprise, and occurs inadvertently through the process of transference.

6   *Informational power*: the accumulation of knowledge has long since been regarded as powerful; Sir Francis Bacon's dictum ([1597] 1985) 'For also knowledge itself is power' in the information age of the

twenty-first century appears to be very apposite; today vast stores of readily available knowledge are contained both in 'hard' form and on the internet, leading to the supposition that there has been a general empowerment of the citizen; however, empowerment depends on access to these resources and the social capital to filter and apply the knowledge once obtained; in therapy, knowledge and the parameters in which that knowledge is delivered are controlled substantially by the therapist.

Disseminated power

Locating power beyond the attributes of the individual and his/her symbolic interaction with others means looking at groupings of individuals. For Michel Foucault (1971; 1973; 1980), power pervades all areas of social life and alters its site and potency over time. Foucault uses the analogy of blood flowing through the body, entering every nook and cranny through a network of large vessels and capillaries. The aorta is filled with large amounts of blood which is then squeezed and sucked into all other organs.

Capillary-like, power is dispersed in society among groups of people (the organs) which are awarded (squeezed into them) or grab (they suck it in) power. Power is diffused and factionalized, is thrust upon groups but it is also 'enjoyed' by them. The professions of medicine and law have been given powers by the state, *and* have purposefully striven to expand their power. This they have done for noble (altruism; justice) and ignoble reasons (greater financial rewards; higher social status). Similarly, the enterprise of therapy is engaged in the squeeze and suck process of power attainment. It has declared its professionalism and works with governments and over-arching regulatory bodies in order to enjoy power.

Foucault, updating the premise of Francis Bacon that 'knowledge is power', argues that certain privileged groups in society (for example, medicine and law) have manufactured their own knowledge in order to authenticate and augment their power. What these groups can then infer is that *their* knowledge is 'truth'. The dispersal of this truth within and across society reinforces the prestige of its purveyors. Administrative apparatus and technical attachments, along with the knowledge, result in a mutually sustaining circle of 'truthful' knowledge and power (Racevskis 1999). The enterprise of therapy has its representative agencies, theories, interpersonal interventions, and boxes of tissues.

An understanding of Foucault's circle of knowledge and power has surprising and counter-intuitive consequences. If social groups can create their own knowledge and set up the conditions under which that knowledge is considered to be correct and comprehensive (that is, a discourse consisting of institutions, tools, and language), then illness is necessary for the continuation of medicine; hearing impairment for audiology; illiteracy and innumeracy for school-teaching; criminality for the police; and misery for therapy. Without one, the other has no justification for its existence.

So, for Foucault, all knowledge is arbitrary and utilitarian. That is, far from knowledge being factual and having both purpose 'in itself' and possible practical application, it is contrived for the specific purpose of giving particular groups power. Moreover, power is lost and won in a never-ending negotiated and renegotiated frenzy of brokerage between groups and as new groups emerge and others wane. Foucault's 'archaeology of knowledge', as he called his academic project, seemed to render impotent the notion of structural power.

Structured power

The stucturalist argument is that there is a framework in society which supplies social identities such as economic class, gender, ethnicity, wealth, and occupation, and these identities have drastic effects on the lives of individuals. Power is a pivotal part of structured society. How much power individuals have to influence society and their personal lives will depend on where they are located in the social structure.

The elites (social classes, or castes) who occupy the top stratum of the structure and command the most important of those institutions in terms of wealth generation, political hegemony, military might, and cultural colonization, produce society's norms, mores and laws. Of course, argue the structuralists, these norms, mores, and laws favour the elites, and sustain their power base in society.

Certainly, if the 'postmodern' stage has been reached in social development, then the old stucturalist position that power is centralized no longer fits. People, even as individuals, have the power to construct their own lives through consumer 'life-style' choices along with the educational and employment opportunities that liberal Western culture affords. But there is a glaring problem with accepting that structuralism has been debunked. Globalization would appear to have *increased*, not decreased, the centralization of power, although the composition of the elites has mutated.

In global society, the principal harbingers and executors of social power are no longer the narrow bunch of elites who were the 'owners of the means of production' as Marxist analyses of nineteenth- and twentieth-century capitalism argued. While the 'owners of the means of production' had a common goal, albeit a loose one, which was to maximize profits within a capitalist mode of economic production, the elites now have a conglomeration of interests. Today the elites have widened their membership, and 'ownership' includes not just financial acumen, but the ability to disseminate widely particular cultural values, and to intimidate through force or the threat of force.

The principal elites in global society are: transnational corporate owners, managers, and senior share-holders; the executors of world financial centres and institutions (the World Bank; the International Monetary Fund); political and military leaders from the wealthiest countries; and the operators of worldwide electronic media and communication networks; the senior members of the United Nations, especially those who are on the Security Council. However, there is a subsidiary group of elites who exercise power locally or internationally: organized crime bosses (especially those who run the mafia, triads, tong, and yakuza); and leaders of environmental groups (for example, Greenpeace), health rights (in particular the World Health Organization, but also hundreds of health NGOs, and human rights groups (for example, Amnesty International).

Virtually all the principal and subsidiary groups are still directly or indirectly, legally or illegally, sponsoring the globalization of capitalism along with its iniquitous social configurations. The exceptions are: terrorist groups, many of whom (for example, the internationalized al-Qaeda; the Maoist Communist Party of Nepal; Shining Path of Peru; the Farc of Colombia) have gained a position of power (in the sense of having a significant membership either worldwide or locally, and by threatening to destabilize their target countries) through campaigning for the overthrow of global (Western) capitalism and its cultural features; environmentalists, some of whom are avowedly anti-capitalist and/or anti-globalization (for example, GMwatch; the Rainforest Action Network; Environmental Working Group; EarthFirst).

An African at risk daily from malnutrition, mutilation, and murder in the Sudanese region of Darfur has little social power compared to the Western Chief Executive of a multi-billion US$ transnational media, bio-chemical, armaments, or petroleum corporation. Moreover, the international inequities are replicated intra-nationally.

Bethan Thomas and Daniel Dorling (2007), with their 'atlas of social identity' have illustrated the clear wealth, health, educational, and age divisions in Britain based on geography. They conclude that from 'cradle to grave' life chances are dictated by location. Health, life-span, and educational and employment success depend on whether or not a person is born and continues to reside in an advantaged or disadvantaged region.

The proponents of globalization consider the spread of the 'free trade' trading system based on Western-style capitalism, Western liberal-democratic and consumerist freedoms to be not only economically but morally justifiable. It will make everyone better off financially, and thereby improve the quality of life for all (Legrain 2003). To begin with, however, this trading system is anything but free or freeing. It is highly structured. Social divisions are shifting, with gender and social class between nations becoming more pronounced than within nations (Perrons 2004). There are massive international and intra-national inequalities in education, employment, wealth, living conditions, health, and life-span. Already globalization contains protected markets, trade barriers, and economic blocs, and these are becoming more common.

Corporate power

Global corporations are the power-brokers of global society. They have immense power and abuse it immensely. For Robert Hare, an expert on psychopathic behaviour, if corporations were people, they would be psychopaths. Corporations, driven by profit, are unconcerned about the seriously negative consequences of their business (for example, the exploitation of already impoverished workers; pollution and global warming). Concern expressed by corporations about these ill-effects is only at a superficial level compassionate and magnanimous (Hare, cited in Bakan 2004).

Here are some examples of corporate psychopathy. Vandana Shiva, physicist and ecologist, in her 2000 Reith Lecture for the BBC (Shiva 2000) entitled 'Poverty and Globalisation' reported on what she described as an 'epidemic' of suicides among farmers in the Punjab, India. Once the most prosperous agricultural region in India, social disaster there has followed ecological disaster. The heavy use of expensive pesticides, due to the trading demands of global capitalism, has not only caused huge debts to mount up among the farming community but also wiped out the natural fauna and created vast stretches of waterlogged land.

Journalists from the British newspaper *The Observer*, in 2006 investigated allegations about the treatment of workers at a clothing factory in Cambodia that supplied some of Britain's leading high street retailers. The majority of workers they met stated that the environment in the factory was too hot and polluted with chemicals (Mathiason and Aglionby 2006).

A six-year investigation by Greenpeace (2006) alleged that some of the largest food companies and commodity traders were responsible for encouraging the illegal destruction of the Amazon rainforest. Virgin forest was being cleared for soya crops to be grown which are then used to feed animals slaughtered to feed European fast-food consumers (mention was made of McDonald's 'chicken McNuggets').

Moreover, Naomi Klein (2007) argues that global corporate capitalism actually *thrives on* crises. For Klein, 'disaster capitalism' makes huge profits from hurricanes, terrorism, tsunamis, civil unrest, and wars. When the population is in 'shock' from a disaster, this presents global corporations with market opportunities because the masses are more willing to accept radical free-market reforms.

John Pilger (2007) in his film *War on Democracy* has pointed to the human rights abuses in Latin America that have been supported by US governments in order to ensure corporate power endures. As pre-eminent linguist and social critic Noam Chomsky (2007) comments, it is the underdeveloped countries that are expected to follow the rules of free trade. When they get into debt by doing so (and they inevitably do because the global market is skewed for the benefit of Western (especially US but also European) elites, then the World Bank and the International Monetary Fund force them to close schools and hospitals. This for Chomsky is cultural and economic hegemonization of global society, which the USA will protect and advance with military intervention when necessary. That is, control by the global elites for the global elites is enacted through hegemony and militarism.

For George Monbiot (2007), global corporations have become so powerful they now threaten the foundations of democratic government and the continued survival of the earth. What he argues is that Western governments are collaborating in their own downfall because they are ceding their power (and therefore the power of the electorate) to these corporations. He accepts the need for globalized trade and a level of industrialization that sustains that trade, but only if it is policed to ensure that ecological disaster is averted and democracy is regained.

Control

Structuralists, therefore, disagree fundamentally with Foucault's proposition that power is distributed for a multitude of groups at all levels of society to 'enjoy'. The power of the global elites for the structuralists is in part achieved through stark exhibitions of power (such as actions by police and courts, and military expeditions). But what is much more pervasive and persuasive than categorical coercion is the myriad of everyday informal networks and interaction, perhaps underwritten by political constitutions and social contracts, which lead to compliance. People are socialized into accepting the tenets and vagaries of a social system through fear of condemnation by the 'agencies of social control', but more effectively by the positive and negative messages disseminated by friends, family, peers, and the media.

These control measures for the most part work well. However, individual states risk disintegration because of civil war, famine, and ecological catastrophe and economic collapse, as well as when large areas of their territory are in the hands of mafia and drug gangs, or terrorists. The Fund for Peace's Conflict Assessment System Tool for 2006 recorded that states most susceptible to failure are: Democratic Republic of the Congo, Côte d'Ivoire, Sudan, Iraq, Zimbabwe, Chad, Somalia, Haiti, Pakistan, and Afghanistan (Fund for Peace 2007).

Post-liberalism

However, Ulrich Beck (1992) argues that 'risk' has become intrinsic to public and business strategies. Within many spheres in society (for example, health, political, employment, and military) 'risk prevention' and 'risk reduction' policies are rife, and there is a plethora of organizations specializing purely in risk. Alongside the culture of risk, there has been a shift in the culture of control.

In the West, since the 1980s a new social contract of rights and responsibilities has been promulgated to help smooth the progress of globalization. People are offered greater freedoms to consume but as a consequence have to be convinced to take on greater responsibility for their communities and themselves. Just prior to the end of Tony Blair's term of office as British Prime Minister, he attempted to instil yet another such social contract (this time concerning health, education, and policing) between citizens and the state (Wintour 2006).

Nikolas Rose (2000) points out that the 'good citizen' has become one who self-regulates and is then rewarded with further rights. The 'bad citizen' (that is one who does not self-regulate) is not just punished but demonized. That is, in what I have termed 'post-liberal' society, the 'bad citizen' becomes susceptible to the discourse of risk thinking, risk management, and the technologies of risk assessment and control (Morrall 2000, 2006b). Defaulting on the responsibilities of the new social contract invites literal or virtual social exclusion. Those targeted for demonization range from the 'dangerous classes' (paedophiles, criminal recidivists, prostitutes, noisy neighbours, the severely mentally ill, and psychopaths) to the 'pathetic classes' (the fat, indolent, drinkers, smokers, and self-harmers).

Therapy in control

John McLeod (2003) offers examples of the therapist's evident connivance with naked social control. These are: when therapists have been referred clients from the courts or work within the prison system, dealing with such misdemeanours as drug or alcohol abuse, and sex offending; universities hire therapists to service the psychological needs of their students, and thereby reduce the number who leave before completing their studies; many large employers have on their payroll therapists to deal with stress/anxiety in the workplace, but also to assist in 'exit strategies' when employees are perceived as unfit to continue in that occupation; the collusion between therapy and psychiatry, with the latter having state-instituted powers of detention and enforced treatment.

Clothed social control is enacted through the 'distortion' of communication (Malhotra 1987; Habermas 1970, 1972). Communicative patterns are encouraged by the elites for the purpose of mystifying underlying exploitations. Through the institutions of education, health, law, and media, the 'hidden agenda' of the elites is manipulating communication. What appears to be the 'right' way of communicating has submerged within it the preferences of the elites. The underlying messages are that materialism, the work ethic, social hierarchies, and personal success and self-improvement, are manifestly normal and natural.

Therapy also indulges in the deliverance of discreet social control. At the start of any therapy session, there are veiled and compelling assumptions about acceptable (to the elites) human performance. The therapeutic discourse essentially replicates these assumptions, and in doing so buttresses the globalization of structural inequalities.

The overt message from therapy is that clients and their private troubles are not abnormal or unusual. But, as Kenneth Gergen (1992) suggests that within each therapy session, and throughout the literature of therapy, the hidden message is that clients have a 'mental deficit'. For Gergen, the therapeutic relationship is a lesson in inferiority for the client and an exhibition of superiority for the therapist.

So, the therapist as agent of social control is sometimes naked and sometimes clothed. Furthermore, therapy performs the social function of filling the social gap between self-regulation and demonization. That is, in post-liberal society, it is therapy that offers the citizen the mechanisms and principles for self-regulation, but if this fails, then more prominent agencies of social control step in.

Crockery, stomping, and chocolate

For example, Heather is a highly self-controlled person for most of the time. If she breaks any social rules, regardless of how minor, she becomes very emotionally distraught and vociferously apologetic. However, sometimes her excessive self-control has a catastrophic failing. When this happens Heather may deliberately and emphatically break another social rule (for example, by binge-drinking to the point of total intoxication, or becoming sexually unconstrained and/or unfaithful), or fly into a Hot Lips Houlihan-type 'red-mist' rage (which might lead to crockery throwing, foot-stomping, or screeching demands such as 'Give me chocolate!'). Attempts by Len to try to help Heather manage her too-controlled and out-of-control performances were largely ineffective. His mixture of psychodynamic searching for childhood causes of her control imbalance, humanistic listening to whatever she said was upsetting her, cognitively reasoning about the illogicality of her reactions, and behavioural rewards when her behaviour matched more exactly the stimulus, were neither capably executed nor welcomed.

More adept and prolonged therapeutic input may have produced better results. But success would only occur if Heather conceded that she had a problem with her self-control, a problem which meant that the tight reins she held on her emotions were always likely to suddenly give way in moments of intense anxiety. There is always the risk that the release of the reins could result in an extreme over-reaction and involve post-liberal demonic behaviour, thereby alerting the foremost agencies of social control such as the police or psychiatry.

Disempowerment

Therapy is abusive, according to some who have been involved directly with it, because it uses its power in such a way as to emasculate those who come to it for help with psychological distress. A word from the ex-therapist turned trouble-maker and cynic Jeffrey Masson:

> The structure of psychotherapy is such that no matter how kindly a person is, when that person becomes a therapist, he or she is engaged in acts that are bound to diminish the dignity, autonomy, and freedom of the person who comes for help.
>
> (Masson 1990: 25)

Throughout his training, Masson records he was beset with doubts, asking such searching questions as: Did therapy make sense?; Is therapy helpful?;

Is the therapist any better than the clients at dealing with psychological distress or those who have had no training in therapy?

This line of questioning, however, I would describe as 'healthy scepticism' not cynicism. These are laudable questions that all students of therapy should ask. If the conclusion from asking these questions is that the therapist and the therapy are not what they purport to be, then to continue to conduct therapy is to be abusive because it is illusionary, exploitative, and disempowering.

Yvonne Bates, along with other contributors to her book *Shouldn't I Be Feeling Better By Now?* (2006), remained sceptical and not cynical. That is, unlike Masson, they are not 'therapy bashers'. What they state they wish to do is to furnish a mature and rigorous debate about the nature of therapy to both therapists and clients.

The contribution of Bates et al. to such a debate reveals serious short-comings in the therapeutic enterprise's quest to empower. For example, they comment that whenever clients criticize their experiences of therapy, the response from therapists tends to be to imply that they were unlucky, or that negativity is an element of their emotional condition. Such rationalizations displace the need for the necessary occupational introspection which would improve therapy. Moreover, Bates asks pointedly:

> Could this tendency be blinding us to the possibility that therapy has many under-examined assumptions masquerading as proven facts, some of which could be exceedingly dangerous or even *abusive*? [emphasis added]
>
> (Bates 2006: viii)

Bates et al. recommend that clients should be informed of the risks at the very start of their engagement in the therapeutic process. It is possible that the client will completely break down emotionally, and lose any self-confidence they brought with them into therapy. Therapy may be contra-indicated with certain forms of psychological distress (for example, post-traumatic stress disorder). Or 'facts' about a client's personal history may be invented as in 'false-memory syndrome' whereby sexual abuse that has supposed to have taken place has been proven not to have done so. Furthermore, the notions of 'personal power', 'non-directiveness', and 'emancipation' within therapy are very misleading. Therapies that claim these attributes are extremely manipulative. Nods or grunts by therapist give signals of approval or disapproval. This is especially the case if the advocator of personal power, non-directiveness and emancipation is a guru in his/her field (as Carl Rogers certainly was when he formulated his humanistic therapy). Up-front advice-giving is much more recommendable ethically. Avoiding gurus is also recommended if the goal is to become empowered.

But, such honesty and 'informed consent' would demystify the power of therapy, and disclose the dependence that it creates in its clients rather than independence. However, Bates et al. report that the reply from therapy to the suggestion for such candidness is that this cannot be accomplished easily as there is no way of knowing how the process and content of the therapy will unfold, and therefore the risks are unknowable. However, such uncertainty exacerbates the power asymmetry within therapy (Pilgrim 1997). The therapist has power, is in control, and the client is exposed to abuse.

Sickness

Another way in which the therapeutic enterprise controls human performance is through the 'sick role'. Being ill for the structural functionalist Talcott Parsons (1951) is not just about how micro-organisms, neoplasms, disability, or physical and psychological trauma affect the body. Illness is regarded by society as a form of deviance and has to be regulated so that society can operate properly. Too much illness would be socially dysfunctional because the economic system would not be serviced, and there would be an unsustainable demand on health and welfare services.

For Parsons, there has to be a formula for allowing a certain amount of 'legitimate' sickness. This formula is a 'social contract' between ill people and the medical profession, which represents the interests of society as a whole. The medical profession is given social power to control access to the sick role, and those designated legitimately ill are given a set of liberties as well as liabilities.

Medicine as agency of social control

Medicine, therefore, has become an agency of social control. But for Parsons this form of social control benefits the whole of society not (only) the elites. Medical practitioners contribute positively to the smooth running of that society through their beneficent interventions with patients, and as agents of social control. However, if the society in which they operate is engulfed by globalization (and most if not all are), then sick role is *de facto* advantaging those already powerful.

The specific way in which the social contract of the sick role functions is though certification. Although self-certification for the initial stage of a period of illness has become standard practice for employees in many

Western industries, medical permission to be away from work for a lengthy period in the main remains mandatory. When an individual is given permission by a medical practitioner to enter into the sick role, he/she (reclassified as a 'patient') is accorded a collection of social privileges together with a number of social obligations (see Table 5.1). The patient is given the right to stay off work, and has exemption from family responsibilities. Moreover, society confers on the patient the right of not being blamed for his/her sickness. His/her duty, however, is to assist in the smooth functioning of society by being motivated to get well.

Table 5.1 Being sick

The sick person	The doctor
Rights of the sick person	*Rights of the doctor*
1. Exemption from role obligations	1. Controls entry to sick role
2. Exemption from responsibility for illness	2. Granted access to intimate information and examination
	3. Professional autonomy and dominance
Obligations of the sick person	*Obligations of the doctor*
1. Must be motivated to get well	1. Acts in accordance with the health needs of the patient
2. Seeks help from and co-operates with doctor	2. Follows the rules of professional conduct
	3. Uses a high degree of expertise and knowledge
	4. Remains objective and emotionally detached

Source: After Parsons (1951)

Medical practitioners also have a set of social privileges and burdens. The profession of medicine is awarded the right to be the paramount agency in controlling access to the sick role, and receives high status and remuneration for doing so. Furthermore, medical practitioners are given social licence to probe the patient's orifices, emotions, and lifestyle.

The socially bestowed obligations of the medical profession are: to always have the health interests of the patient at heart when delivering treatment; adherence to stringent guidelines for practice, which are formulated by the profession itself; to undergo lengthy and rigorous (scientific) training, which is also formulated by the medical profession; and to act impartially and impersonally.

Other health disciplines, such as pharmacy and nursing, and therapists who are employed directly in the health service (for example, by general practitioners), are at times delegated this social task of controlling sickness. Therapists, apart from direct delegation by medical practitioners, have an indirect but expanding role in controlling sickness, which is expanding.

Parsons did not believe that his model of sick role could be found in every case of illness, or that medical practitioners and their patients performed consistently in their respective roles. What he presented was an 'ideal type': a model that could be used to try to understand a particular social phenomenon (in this case, sickness), without it answering all of the concerns relating to that phenomenon or removing the possibility of alternative understandings.

But there are glaring faults with Parson's model. Realistically, many people are not able to take advantage of their rights when sick. Women who are in paid employment and become ill still tend to have to care for their children and hence cannot easily 'take to their beds'. Whilst Parson's sick role may be an appropriate way of describing what occurs in acute illness, when people suffer from chronic illness it is less likely that their social obligations will be met. For example, it is symptomatic of depression that the sufferer will not be motivated to get well. Moreover, certain diseases are socially stigmatized (for example, AIDS and alcoholism). Here the individual is blamed for contracting the condition. That is, with these conditions the right not to be held accountable for contracting the illness is not afforded. Medical practitioners also may not always be working directly for the benefit of their patients. Some are 'in it for the money', others are incompetent or abusive, and a few are murderous (Morrall 2006a). Also, Parsons' conceptualization of the patient is one of 'passivity'. In today's Western health systems (and increasingly developing and underdeveloped countries that may be involved with, for example, the empowerment policies of the World Health Organization) emphasis is placed on patient 'activity'.

Therapy as an agency of social control

Moreover, other disciplines have been recruited to the administration of sickness, including therapy. That is, there is an overlap between the social status of 'being sick' and 'being in therapy'. The overlap may be complete if being in therapy is regarded as a form of sickness, as it is occasionally formally but more often it is inferred. As with other forms of sickness, the personal dysfunction that brings a client to therapy has the same potential to harm the functioning of society as physical and psychological disorders that are treated medically. This overlap between medicine and therapy is patent when general practitioners refer or delegate their patients to therapists (or psychologists), and when psychiatrists and psychiatric nurses indulge in talking treatments. In these circumstances the enterprise of therapy is unavoidably acting as agency of social control.

There are, however, important caveats to this claim that therapy is an agency of social control within the sick role (see Table 5.2). While the client may be encouraged to attend therapy by an employer, it is not compulsory in the way that visiting a medical practitioner is when sickness strikes. However, it may be considered by the employer a deviation from the obligations of the sick role if the patient refuses to undergo therapy. The client, unlike the patient, is usually expected to 'own' the problem that has necessitated therapy. But there is within therapy what I have termed the 'paradox of responsibility'. On the one hand, the client blaming someone else (for example, partner or parent) for how he/she feels, thinks, or behaves is certainly for humanist and cognitive-behavioural therapists deemed disempowering. On the other hand, therapy generally doesn't propose the idea that the client is culpable for his/her plight because this is also deemed disempowering.

Table 5.2 Being in therapy

The client	The therapist
Rights of the client	*Rights of the therapist*
1. Exemption from role obligations	1. Controls entry to sick role by proxy/ incidentally
2. Paradox of client's responsibility for his/her personal problems (ownership without blame)	2. Granted access to intimate information
	3. Drive towards professional autonomy and dominance
Obligations of the client	*Obligations of the therapist*
1. Motivated as a key factor	1. Expected to act in accordance with the emotional needs of the patient
2. Seeks technical help (voluntarily in the main but increasingly becoming formalized) from therapist	2. Expected to follow the rules of professional conduct
	3. Expected to have high degree of expertise and knowledge
	4. Remains emotionally engaged

Summary

Social power infiltrates all social situation and relationships, including therapy. Power accumulates, however, in certain parts of society. It may be expropriated by the ruling elites, or disseminated to disparate social groupings. Uncontrolled power can pervert society, encouraging the disavowal of human rights. But the exertion of power by the state and other social institutions is also indispensable for the perpetuation of society, and for the protection of susceptible groups. Without significant restraining mechanisms, society would disintegrate, leaving only anarchy and barbarism. The sick role is one means by which society controls deviancy to aid social constancy *and* vulnerable people (the sick). Therapy has become implicated in social control. Social control is part of what therapists do and what therapy represents.

Nick Totton (2006) believes that therapists should willingly and actively enter politics. For him an individual's psychological distress cannot be disconnected from social power. That is, the cause of much of human suffering has social origins. Furthermore, Totton argues that the way to redress the disproportionate allocation of power within the therapeutic relationship is to 'place it dead centre'. That is, resolution to the problems of power should be sought through negotiation between the therapist and the client. Certainly, this is an honest and open strategy that is recommended by Totton.

However, social power is so deeply imbedded within therapy, and people in conditions of psychological distress are so vulnerable, that the 'Totton Plan' may, notwithstanding its good intentions and meticulous intellectualization, be as effective/ineffective as the Freudian proposal that resolution of internal conflicts will assist social evolution, the commitment of humanist therapists to a 'quiet revolution', or the crusade by cognitive-behaviourists for pandemic bliss.

What Monbiot (2004) wants is authentic global democracy. For Monbiot, power should be given to people with the creation of a world parliament. The globalization of society requires a globalized solution to globally orchestrated and globally structured abuses.

Perhaps the most insidious aspect of abuse by therapy, however, is what Masson calls the 'corruption of friendship'. The client is offered a relationship that may appear to be a friendship, in that he or she is encouraged to share his or her closest secrets and feelings, but that is in reality a false friendship. The relationship between therapist and client, Masson points out, is a professional one, based on an inequality in power. Heather and Len's relationship contained the inverse of this falsehood. He abused her by dispensing therapy (albeit coarsely) along with friendship. She abused him by accepting therapy (albeit begrudgingly) along with friendship.

CHAPTER 6

Infectious

Professions
Medicalization
Therapyitis

Therapy is infectious. The therapeutic enterprise is spreading plague-like across Western society and is rapidly contaminating the rest of global society.

Since the inception of therapy, professionalization has been its main occupational strategy (House 2003). The enterprise of therapy is presently fostering its campaign to emulate law, and especially medicine, through certification and registration. But caution is recommended about this drive to become a profession. It may be that a non-professional status is a better choice as better option for therapy, for its clients, and for society. Although the cultural infiltration of professions such as medicine has flourished, this has not been without a serious down-side. Similarly, the budding cultural infiltration of therapy has a dangerous spin-off.

Professionalization will promulgate the progress of the therapy pandemic. But too much therapy runs the risk of becoming poisonous in a comparable way to the disabling effect of too much medicine. That is, therapyitis (Morrall 2007a) undermines the individual's ability to take care of his/her psychological distress and reduces public issues to private troubles just as 'medicalization' has thwarted the individual's facility to manage his/her health care and allowed the state to downgrade its responsibility for socially created disease.

It is to be expected that therapy would try to emulate medicine. Therapy emerged at the turn of the twentieth century from the intellectual and practical pursuits of a medical man (Sigmund Freud). Although some 'collaborators' continued to supply the medical sub-speciality of psychiatry with the knowledge and skills derived from their expanding therapeutic discourse, therapy and medicine descended into a century of competitive enmity. However, while neither has been victorious in this particular hundred-year-war, as with the enmity between the French and English, an uneasy armistice has broken out. Therapy and medicine are progressively more in cahoots with each other, although again as with the French and English, suspicion and distaste linger. Increasingly, therapy, especially the 'quick-fix' variety, is being advocated as an adjunct to medical intervention.

Heather is also infectious. The 'Hyde' of her dichotomous 'Dr Jekyll and Mr Hyde' performance can be detrimental to the health of others. For those who become addicted to the toxic concoction of neediness, ferocity, and sultriness (as did Len), then mind and body homeostasis is likely to be disrupted severely.

However, therapy and Heather are infectious in the positive as well as negative meaning of the term. As with 'infectious laughter' and 'infectious optimism', Heather, when being bright and buoyant, is beguiling, and therapy, when selling satisfaction and self-actualization, is seductive.

Professions

Therapy is an immature discipline. Like the adolescent period in human development, therapy is weighed down by uncertainties over identity and performance, and while rehearsing the appropriate ways of adulthood, childishness and ungainliness spurt through the protective sheath of bravado.

Maturity is the expected outcome of adolescence. But for some people it is either late in coming or never arrives, and 'inappropriate' behaviour persists. The same may be the fate of therapy. Therapy may remain with the unedifying swagger of a teenage occupation, proclaiming its virility and discernment but reaching old age without ever growing up to accept both its occupational limitations and responsibilities. Medicine, on the other hand, has entered adulthood. That is, doctors and their agencies are engaged with social suffering (the prime example is *Médecins Sans Frontières*), and have realized the limits of medicine and its detrimental propensity.

Heather has the performance swings of the adolescent. She can be juvenile in her reactions to events or comments, especially those that she determines as threats to her 'self'. Nevertheless, she is capable of the most magnanimous of acts, the highest moral positioning, and perspicacity way beyond her life's experience. Contrarily, it may be that the mixture of childishness and adultness is what gives Heather the aura she is famed for. Bizarrely, it may also be what keeps Len, her barefoot therapist, so hooked on his quest to help settle her psychological impasses, many of which ironically are intertwined with her child–adult oscillations.

Equally, regardless of its troubling conflicts, lotteries and rivalries, arrogance, selfishness, abusiveness, and infectiousness, therapy is incredibly alluring. For clients of therapy, there is an equivalent of the sensual pay-off afforded Len for the frustrations and fearfulness he suffers with Heather. Just as Heather dangles her womanly charms to entice Len into contests of psychological wrestling (and the occasional arm-rustling match), so therapy seduces its clients with evocations of attainment and/or contentment.

But therapy does *want* to be all grown-up. That is, a fully-fledged professional status is either openly avowed or implicitly aspired to by therapists and their organizations. But it is nowhere near that goal as yet. Worse still, there appears to be little understanding by therapists of what a profession in reality is, and of what is happening in the world of work that might indicate a more appropriate occupational route than professionalization.

Work in a changing world

Globalization is transforming work. Service industries have largely replaced manufacturing industries in the West. The pace of industrialization in developing countries (in particular China and India) is incredibly fast. 'Outsourcing' of work is common practice depending on where in the world advantageous labour markets (particularly in underdeveloped countries which are likely to have minimal health and safety regulations, low wages, little unionization, and few rules about hiring and firing) can be found. Most products (from computers to cars) are made up of components manufactured in several countries. Although government departments remain major employers, there has been a move by the state in many countries to be the purchaser rather than provider of services. Those services that the state still directly provides have been opened up to internal market economics. 'Flexible' work patterns abound (characterized by low pay and unsocial hours), and linked to flexibility is the feminization of the workforce (that is, more women in employment than men).

But, while people in employment continue to have a substantial part of their lives taken up by their work, and the retirement age in Western countries is rising, much of the world's adult population is under-employed, underpaid, or unemployed. In 2006, there were 200 million unemployed people and 1.37 billion people who were in 'work poverty' earning less than US$2 per day (United Nations 2007). Moreover, social strife or political incompetence can result in periods of the sudden and severe loss of employment opportunities. For example, an economic crisis in Zimbabwe, fuelled by government decisions concerning the ownership of land in 2000 and subsequent attempts to diminish informal trading, had the consequence of increasing the unemployment rate to 80 per cent (Central Intelligence Agency 2007).

In such a dynamic and globalized work (and non-work) environment, the professions are inevitably affected. The elevated occupational position of established professions such as law and medicine may not be maintained, just as previous professions (for example, the clergy and school teaching) have become 'de-professionalized'. Moreover, many other occupational groups are emerging and vying for professional status. There is also the possibility that the old demarcations of 'professional' and 'non-professional' (along with those of 'white-collar' and 'blue-collar') will become meaningless because work is mutating so fast, bringing the demise in deference to experts, and/or the professions lose their previous role within society.

Defective definitions

But what is a profession? Defining 'profession' has a long history in sociology, and has been debated interminably to the point of tedium. What follows is an abridged account of the twentieth-century sociological reasoning about professions. The outcome of this review I suggest leaves the version tendered by Eliot Freidson as the most relevant to an analysis of where therapy fits in the occupational hierarchy.

Sociological thinking about professions inherited tautological explanations which relied on criteria supplied by those who regarded themselves already as professionals (namely lawyers, medical practitioners, and clerics). Professional 'traits' were identified by these informants (altruism;

specialized knowledge; lengthy training; monopoly over a field of practice; and self-regulation). Then along came the functionalist approach to suggest that occupational groups exhibiting these traits helped the society to operate efficiently: the profession of medicine controlled entry into the sick role; the profession of law arbitrated justice.

But what was glaringly omitted in these early theories was reference to social power. Society gave the professionals power and they in turn exercised that power. For example, feminists argued that patriarchy in society was replicated in the professions: men occupied and ruled the professions. Therapy also suffers from patriarchal inequity. Women outnumber men as therapists and as clients, and women can be found in the lexicon of therapy gurus (for example, Melanie Klein and Hanna Segal). But the founding gurus of therapy were men, and, as with nursing, men remain more visible within therapy academia and the higher echelons of the therapeutic enterprise.

Marxists couldn't make up their minds as to whether or not professionals were on the side of the proletariat (and therefore subjugated), in league with the bourgeoisie (and hence exploitative), or in a transitory position between the two. McLeod (2003) points out that most therapists are either from or become 'middle class'. However, unlike the patrons of both law and medicine, most clients of therapy are also from the middle class. Consequently, the allegiance of therapy to either the exploitative or the subjugated is not straightforward.

Postmodernist considerations imply that the professions are not aligned necessarily with any one social class. The power of professionals is much more localized. Power is 'enjoyed' for its own sake (high social status and generous remuneration) rather than directly serving the requirements of the state, although it may do either incidentally or as a requirement of continued support by the state. 'Discursive practices' (i.e. the technologies, procedures, and linguistic styles of a particularly powerful social group) are the central means by which the professions develop and maintain their power (Foucault 1966, 1973). But, for the postmodernists, there is nothing intrinsically 'better' about a profession compared with other occupations. Moreover, the demise in deference towards experts, and the potential for power to evaporate from the established professions and emerge in other occupations as a consequence of the vagaries of consumer preference, could result in the hierarchical position of doctors and lawyers plummeting.

This is the point made by historian Harold Perkin (2000). Perkin points out that human capital has been intensified and demarcated in universities through the setting-up of departments representing a multiplicity of novel academic, technological, scientific, and vocational subjects (therapy being one of them). For Perkin, Western society has reached the age of the 'specialized expert', and specialization is helping to drive globalization. However, observes Perkin, there has also been a deliberate attempts to undermine the professions. British Prime Minister Margaret Thatcher's governments of the later twentieth century in particular attacked the apparent immune social status of doctors, lawyers, school teachers, senior civil servants, scientists not engaged in applied research, and university lecturers (notably sociologists). Hence, for Perkin, the professionals are just as vulnerable to loss of social status (and employment) as any other groups of workers.

The contributions to answering the question 'What is a profession?' by functionalists, Marxists, feminists, postmodernists, and historians are illuminating. But, I suggest, it is only the analysis of the medical profession by Eliot Freidson (1970; 1971; 1988; 1994; 2001) that still has credibility in a global society. Moreover, although committed to the sociology of Max Weber, the continued appositeness of Freidson's approach rests of his incorporation of a range of theoretical insights from other social theorists.

Autonomy and dominance

Freidson's main point was that the professions served primarily themselves rather than their patients or society, and their power was used to guarantee privilege. Genuine professionals (for Freidson, these were primarily law and medicine) realized their power through achieving autonomy over set areas of work and domination over everyone else working in the same field.

Medicine has gained its autonomy and dominance through the deployment of a range of effective tactics over hundreds of years. These include: beating its early competitors (the apothecaries; the butchers; the lay-mid-wives; the herbalists; the priests); political manoeuvrings (aided by the 'cultural affinity' between doctors and those in authority – Thatcher accepted); social closure (re-designing medicine as an exclusive, self-regulated occupation, with its own mystifying discourse); and alignment with science (medicine has adopted science as its epistemological guarantor).

The power of medicine has, however, become diminished – but not destroyed. Medicine still maintains much of its high social status and remuneration, autonomy, and dominance despite managerial intrusion, the popularity of non-scientific and lay health care, the increased sphere of authority and practice given to paramedical disciplines, patient empowerment, and bad press from blundering and malevolent medical practitioners. Doctors may err and murder, but they still are politically astute compared with other health occupations. Moreover, they are served well by their epistemological ally in the present era of revolutionary scientific and technological discovery.

Freidson, surprisingly, is in favour of the professions despite their serious shortcomings, just as I am sympathetic to therapy notwithstanding its fundamental flaws, and Len's devotion to Heather is not diminished despite her deeply daunting 'Hyde'. The motivation of medical strategists has been one primarily of self-interest not altruism, but Freidson seems to accept the functionalist premise that social institutions and their members have a positive purpose in society. While arguing, for example, that medicine's *raison d'être* is not wholly humanitarian, he appreciates that it does contribute constructively to the working of society, and that its practitioners, as with therapists and Heather, do carry out meritorious acts.

Medicalization

But social commentators Ivan Illich, Irving Zola and John McKnight (Illich et al. 1977) take a censorious view of professionals. For them, experts form 'institutional barricades', and from within these barricades experts act as gate-keepers and breed knowledge and practices that serve *their* interests, not those of their customers/patients/clients. Illich and his colleagues regard professionalization not as enabling but disabling for society.

The profession of medicine for Illich (1975) has over-stimulated the health wants of Western society through medicalization. Medicalization is spreading throughout global society, and is doing so all the more successfully because it is encompassing former epistemological enemies. Traditional, complementary, and alternative health care is being scientized and thereby succumbing to medical governance (Morrall 2008).

Bleeding women and irritable men

The medicalization of everyday life in the West is rampant. New syndromes and diseases are discovered (or 'invented') daily. A huge variety of social and personal phenomena are now administrated by the medical enterprise. Menstruation is no longer a natural if unwelcome 'curse', but a medical 'condition' to be regulated. Pre-menstrual tension is not a period of unavoidable (and unmentionable) hormonal imbalance, but a syndrome to be soothed. A large body no longer signifies simply a big appetite or, as in some Asian and African cultures, high social status, but has become a stigmatized disorder in both developed and developing societies. Feeling tired, miserable, and disinterested is not merely a personality trait but is myalgic encephalomyelitis ('chronic fatigue syndrome'), or if during the winter 'seasonal affective disorder'. Being drunk and feckless is no longer a lifestyle choice (albeit a self-destructive one) but 'alcoholism'. Deformity is not the unfortunate by-product of normal birth or untoward mishaps, but an unacceptable physical aberration in a world which venerates the body; any bulge or blemish, absent or superfluous entity, can be removed or replaced to ensure physical perfection. School children are not naughty but have 'attention deficits' or are 'hyperactive'. Idiosyncratic writing and reading is not a learning difficulty but 'dyslexia'. Killing another human may not be murder but 'Munchausens'. Paedophilia is not just a crime but a diagnosable psychiatric illness. Having bombs dropped around you while in the company of your neighbours means that you may contract 'complete mass conflict disorder' rather than just being scared witless. Cantankerous and short-tempered men can now claim to have caught 'irritable male syndrome'.

Individualizing social problems

Sociologists, frequently invoking the polemical stance of Illich, have been consistently critical of medicalization (the term is mostly used pejoratively). Apart from the obvious 'social control' aspects in medical practice (which sustain the status quo and therefore benefit the powerful elites in society), there is an indirect 'control' effect of medicalization that is far more potent. When a doctor treats a patient for an ailment such as bronchitis, heart failure, lung cancer, or mental disorder, the focus of the intervention is on the individual. It is the *individual* who is asked to strip for examination, it is his/her blood that is sent to the laboratory for investigation, and to whom medication is supplied or on whom surgery performed. Many (if not all) serious illnesses have social and environmental dimensions, but society is not medicated or surgically readjusted.

The same process happens through therapy. By concentrating exclusively on the patient, the medical practitioner and the therapist are individualizing social problems. That is, medical practice reinforces the very social system that is the source of much disease. Moreover, the responsibility of the state to change society is diminished while doctors carry out remedial interventions on individuals.

Doctors against medicalization

But the medical profession is aware of the pitfalls of its own exuberance, although they are tempted to blame others. The journal *Public Library of Science Medicine* (2006) published eleven articles by US and British medical experts. The claim was made in these articles that pharmaceutical corporations were 'diseasemongering'. Pharmaceutical corporations were inventing new disorders, or whenever the medical profession did so itself, they were quick to understand the profits to be made in encouraging the authenticity of such discoveries and subsequently pressurized doctors to offer drug treatments. British general practitioner Michael Fitzpatrick (2000) in his book *The Tyranny of Health* writes that the risks from disease are being exaggerated by politicians and thereby causing high levels of anxiety among his patients. Patients demand treatments when they are healthy not diseased, argues Fitzpatrick. In a more mature understanding of medical complicity (that is, one that doesn't shift the blame onto corporations, governments, or consumers) Richard Smith (2002), editor of the *British Medical Journal*, recommends that all medical students should read Illich's treatise on medicalization. He and journalist Ray Moynihan suggest not only demedicalization but deprofessionalization:

> Perhaps some doctors will now become the pioneers of de-medicalisation. They can hand back power to patients, encourage self care and autonomy, call for better worldwide distribution of simple effective health care, resist the categorisation of life's problem as medical, promote the de-professionalisation of primary care, and help decide which complex services should be available.
>
> (Smith and Moynihan 2002: 860)

Iagotrogenesis

For Illich, the medical establishment has put both the health of individuals and society in jeopardy as a consequence of doctor-inflicted injuries and loss of self-autonomy – what Illich describes as 'iatrogenesis'. Medical intervention, argues Illich, is such a cause of morbidity and mortality it can be viewed as one of the most rapidly spreading epidemics of modern times. A definition more appropriate for today's health systems, I suggest, is that of 'healer-induced harm' whereby the 'healer' is still often a medical practitioner but may now be a nurse, midwife, physiotherapist, audiologist, or therapist, and the 'harm' can be immediate, delayed, short-term, long-term, minimal, major, direct, indirect, localized or globalized.

Illich viewed iatrogenesis in three forms. First, there is *clinical iatrogenesis*. Here Illich is referring to the most obvious negative consequences of medical intervention. These range from the damage done physically and emotionally to patients from medication, surgery, mistakes, and hospitalization (McTaggart 2005). All pharmaceutical products have side-effects (generally the more toxic, the medication the more lethal the by-product), and approximately 5,000 patients in Britain alone are dying from adverse reaction to their prescribed drugs (British Medical Association, cited in Bosely 2006). Known medical errors seriously harm 1.5 million US citizens annually (Roerh 2006), and one in ten patients globally (World Health Organization 2005). Unnecessary operations are on the increase because of the stepping-up of medical liability generating a 'better safe than sorry' mentality among practitioners and insurers (termed 'defensive medicine'); a large landfill site could easily be filled to overflow with the debris from gratuitous laparotomies, biopsies, appendectomies, tonsillectomies, adenoidectomies, episiotomies, gastroectomies, mastectomies, hysterectomies, abortions, caesareans, and aesthetic corrections.

Defensively, the American College of Surgeons state as one of their professional principles:

> No operation should be performed without suitable justification. It is the surgeon's responsibility to perform a careful evaluation, including consultation with others when appropriate, and to recommend operation only when it is the best method of treatment for the patient's problem.
>
> (American College of Surgeons 2006)

Such a proclamation should, certainly by 2006, be redundant. It is akin to the police authorities telling their officers to avoid committing crimes, or transport companies stipulating that their drivers should avoid crashes, or the agencies of therapy advising their practitioners to, as much as possible, not hit their clients.

A century and a half ago, Florence Nightingale had recommended that a hospital should do no harm. But the incidence of disease and death arising not from what one brings into hospital, but from what one catches from being in hospital, is increasing. The hospital-acquired infections methicillin-resistant staphylococcus aureu (MRSA), clostridium difficile, pseudomonas, and Acinetobacter baumannii debilitate and kill hundreds of thousands of patients (civilian and military) across the world.

The equivalent to clinical iatrogenesis within the therapeutic enterprise has an equivalent 'dark underbelly' to the clinical iatrogenesis of medicine. Some therapies do immediate and noticeable (psychological) harm. That is, the side-effect to undergoing some therapies can be more, rather than less, psychological distress (Jarrett 2008).

Second, Illich refers to *social iatrogenesis*, whereby the whole of society becomes dependent on the medical profession. People become addicted to not just medicines but to the medical profession. Furthermore, we look to doctors to sort out out not just our diseases but our interpersonal strife, child-rearing practices, sexual inadequacy, unhappiness, and penalties from lifestyle choices and over-indulgencies. Such dependence, for Illich, has made the medical profession extremely powerful.

Third, Illich posits that clinical iatrogenesis and social iatrogenesis lead to such entrenchment of medical authority in all areas of human life that the individual loses his or her ability to make autonomous judgements. This end-product of medical intrusion into how we organize our lives Illich describes as *cultural iatrogenesis*. Cultural iatrogenesis has incapacitated the individual. He/she is unable to make personal decisions about his/her life, or experience pain, suffering, and death as an inescapable part of existence. Hence humans have become separated from their own humanity, nature, and reality.

Healthism

Robert Crawford has identified, however, a social process that extends substantially the medical intrusiveness into our lives. This he describes as 'healthism' (Crawford 1980). By the 1970s, there was an explosion of commercial and politically sponsored interest in exercise, jogging, diets, vitamins, fitness machines, and anti-stress measures. By the 2000s, healthism had gone much further, bringing an aggressive anti-smoking, anti-alcohol, anti-fat, anti-cholesterol, anti-lazy, pro-fitness, pro-slimness, pro-moderation, and pro-happiness ethic.

The health police, an amalgam of medical practitioners, nurses, disciplines allied to medicine, politicians, and therapists, are patrolling human performance as never before in human history. In the USA, the principal agency for 'protecting the health of all Americans', the Department of Health and Human Services (DHHS), considers large areas of human performance to be its responsibility. For example:

- Coping
- Eating Right
- Drinking
- Sun, Air, Home, Workplace, School
- Exercise and Fitness
- General Wellness and Healthy Lifestyle
- Smoking and Tobacco
- Traveler's Health
- Violence, Abuse, and Neglect

The health police were out in full force in Britain under the government of Tony Blair. During the month of August 2006, people with a disorder of the mind were to be told to get their bodies in order by specially trained 'well-being nurses' who were to help the thousands of already instilled 'health trainers' (Department of Health 2006a). Five days later this advice about becoming physically fit extended to everyone so that the population would be ready for the 2012 Olympics (Department of Health 2006b). Eight days later obese people were targeted for special physical activity measures (Department of Health 2006c). The previous year, the health police had tried to outlaw stilton cheese:

> The centuries-old recipe that gives Stilton, the "king of English cheeses", its distinctive flavour is under threat from the Government's anti-salt campaigners. Cheese makers say they are under pressure to slash levels of salt to meet the Department of Health's targets … But they argue that it plays a key role in the creation of all blue cheeses and that tampering with the recipe could be disastrous … Salt is added partly for taste, partly to drive out moisture and also to slow the development of bacteria.
>
> (Derbyshire 2005)

Crawford's prescient prediction was that normality as well as deviance would become medicalized. Government health departments, the World Health Organization, and the alternative/complementary health bandwagon consider failure to be as healthy as a failure of will. Unhealthiness is now a deviance, healthiness is the model for 'good living', and the healthy are 'good citizens' and the unhealthy are 'bad citizens'. *Healthism*, from the constructionist viewpoint, is part of the consumer culture, stimulated by the pharmaceutical companies, media, fashion industries, and sports/fitness enterprises. Health is procured as a commodity, and has become yet another facet of what both structuralists and postmodernists might agree is 'conspicuous consumption' (Greenhalgh and Wessely 2004).

Therapyitis

Healthism directed towards British psychological improvement is escalating, and has received an enormous boost largely thanks to the prodigious commitment of Lord Richard Layard to tidy up the 'disordered' minds of the public. Layard, an economist and social policy advisor to the British government, is a champion of what he describes as 'evidence-based therapies'. He is in particular a devotee of cognitive-behaviour therapy (CBT). Along with his team from the London School of Economics Centre for Economic Performance's Mental Health Policy Group, Layard has offered a 'new deal' to millions of miserable and agitated Britons (Layard 2006a). Layard's mission to mollify misery and assuage agitation requires, he suggests, 10,000 extra therapists to be employed for the NHS.

Psycho-healthism

'Psycho-healthism' (my term for the proliferation of policies, practices, and commodities designed to advance the psychological well-being of the masses) is also encroaching more and more into the realm of family relationships. *Relate*, the British therapy service, announced in 2006 the opening of what it describes as 'a centre of excellence' in Doncaster for the study of couple and family relationships (*Relate* 2006). The *Relate Institute*, proclaimed by *Relate* to be a centre of excellence, at its inception in 2006 aimed to start training hundreds of couple and family specialists. Courses at the Institute cover such topics as psychodynamic therapy, systemic therapy, psychosexual therapy, couple therapy, sexuality, sexual abuse, mental disorder, research methods.

On the surface, the setting-up of the *Relate Institute* seems a tremendous advance in catering for the needs of adults and children in families where relationships are strained or shattered, and in the promotion of 'healthy' family relationships to prevent straining or shattering in the first place. However, psycho-healthism can also be construed as insidiously disempowering, and considered a virulent form of social engineering. The basis on which laudable Lord Layard and the good burghers of *Relate* make judgements about how individuals should think, feel, and behave (and thereby) is a flawed idealization of human performance born from an uncritical and expedient acceptance of particular 'scientific' data-selected theories. Moreover, it is undemocratic if not verging on dictatorial to unleash thousands of mind-altering emissaries on an unsuspecting public and plunge society further into the therapeutic equivalent of medicalization: therapyitis.

Decrees about deficits in human performance cannot be divorced from the self-interest of those wishing to offer corrective services. For Frank Furedi (2003), an ever-widening definition of psychological distress and the manufacture of a plethora of psychological disorders, along with the preparation of an army of psychological healers prepared to tackle any and all types of distress, here resulted in a 'therapy culture'. There is, therefore, an inflation of the importance of psychological distress and the need for therapeutic intervention. Moreover, no matter how loud and frequently the mantra of self-determination is asserted by therapists, for Furedi, their clients are caught in an emotional Catch-22 by the very fact of receiving help for their personal problems. Furthermore, as with Illich's point about medicalization, therapyitis is not only disabling for the individual but leads to society becoming debilitated.

Consumer demand

Stucturalist sociology views consumers as passive addicts, prey to the exploitative dealers in the production of medicalization and healthism. But medicalization is not all the fault of doctors or executives of health corporations. Although the medical profession and the merchants of healthism stimulate and feed the health market with a never-ending supply of commodities, labels and promises, consumerist lust is excited in part by the public. People *want* pills, potions, yoga and yogurt to be diagnosed, and to believe that a cure for everything will (eventually) be delivered. Interactionist sociology considers consumers as not addicted but free to construct their own values about health and decide for themselves whether or not to buy from the medical and health dealers (given that their social circumstances will circumscribe that freedom). However, the sociology of Anthony Giddens (1986; 1991) shows the reflexive relationship between the addict and the dealer. Each needs the other.

There would seem to be no shortage of dealers in emotional in-touchness and emotionally in-touch addicts. In recognition of the supply–demand symbiosis, research by the Future Foundation (2004) for the British Association for Counselling and Psychotherapy (BACP), reported that therapy has gained mass acceptance among what it describes as the more 'emotionally in-touch' section of the population. In 2006, a new mind publication was produced, and two years later it has survived a viciously competitive market in popular health journals. *Psychologies Magazine* is pandering to an already receptive set of (female) consumers. But, it has such a superlative sales pitch and extensive range of topics that only the most emotionally out-of-touch could resist. Its editor introduces the first edition thus:

> Welcome to *Psychologies*, the first women's magazine that is about what we are really like, not just what we look like. If you are interested in the ways we think, behave, communicate and connect, then this is for you. Whether you want to develop your own potential, or become a better parent, partner or friend, we will bring you the ideas, insights and inspiration to help you do it. We all have more choices and more demands on our time than ever before. In a fast-changing world, the greatest skill we can have is to understand ourselves, and the people around us. With support from experts, who are leaders in the fields of

behaviour, personality, emotions and relationships, we will present practical strategies and mind shifting insights to help you develop that understanding, and to live a richer life.

(Maureen Rice 2006)

The 'experts' who contribute to *Psychologies* include medical practitioners, psychologists, and therapists who cover: psychotherapy; depression; inspiration; miscarriage; mugging; grieving; guilt; overeating; rejection; relationships; jealousy; insecurity; arguments; commitment; anger; alcoholism; cruelty; intimacy; love; abuse; misery; worry; anxiety; sex; violence; and thumb-sucking.

Fast food, fast cars, and fast erections

It is in the interests of therapeutic enterprise to comply with the spread of a competitive, capitalist, consumer culture. Consumerism and therapy both require individualism. The insanity of a global society that gives high prestige to fast food, fast cars, and fast erections, while low priority is given to malnutrition, malaria, and malevolence, is not only accepted but *recommended* by today's more fashionable therapies.

Global capitalism's endorsement of fast food, fast cars, and (drugs for) fast erections, is part of the commodification of life whereby 'natural' human activities (eating, travelling from place-to-place, and having sex) are packaged as special lifestyle choices. Problems with living have also been packaged.

The BACP in 2004 put an advert in a national newspaper headed 'Changing Career? Want to Become a Counsellor?'. The BACP's attempt to encourage new recruits, however, seemed to be based on selling a training directory it produces (which lists hundreds of therapy courses run by training institutes and universities) – for the sum of £19 (US$36). Moreover, the business wing of BACP, BACP Enterprises, publicizes services and products from therapy organizations by advertising these in specialist journals. In 2006, the charges for advertising in the BACP's own journal was, approximately £1,575 (nearly US$3,000). Admittedly, this was for a full-page colour spread.

Whole-being healers and tarot readers

Another stark example of psychological distress becoming a commodity is the multiplicity of provision. I live in a small northern English city, yet we are very generously served by therapy and therapy-type private services. An *ad hoc* review I conducted in 2006 (updated in 2008) of the local telephone business listings and newspapers, public library/cinema leaflet displays, and internet sites, found approximately 60 individual counselling/psychotherapy practitioners and 25 centres/institutes. This is apart from the state-run psychiatric hospital and several clinical units, and a variety of voluntary mental health facilities. Furthermore, there was an array of complementary therapists/therapies (and 40 courses at the local further education college) that either directly or indirectly dealt with psychological distress. Examples are:

Barry, the Whole Being Healing/Healer therapist

Sarah, fully qualified life coach (also runs courses in total relaxation and meditation and is a chartered accountant)

The Human Givens Centre (attendance at which will resolve conflict, control anger, lift depression, reduce anxiety, stop phobias, lessen stress, eliminate panic attacks, increase self-confidence, lower emotional arousal, and relieve pain)

Ming Imperial Herbal Inn Healing (herbs for arthritis, infertility, bloating, fibroids, menopause, slimming, impotence, prostatitis, depression, insomnia, migraine, eczema, acne, psoriasis, alopecia, haemorrhoids, and 'many more')

Yoga (for beginners, revisers, and the pregnant)

Buddhist Meditation

Reflexology (helping with depression, as well as: acne; asthma; colds; depression; eczema; heartburn; insomnia; migraine; allergies; shoulder pain; constipation; diverticulitis; hay fever; indigestion; menopause; neck problems; and whiplash)

Practical Philosophy (to find rest for an over-active mind; connect with the joy of living; discover the real self, a larger view of the world, and purpose of life)

Hypnosis Workshops/Luminous Life Hypnotherapy (for low self-esteem, grief, depression and regression, as well as obesity and smoking)

Divorce Recovery Workshop

Meditation

Reiki

Seichem

Indian Head Massage

Eastern Head Massage

At Ease Therapies

Kinesiology

Aromatherapy

Holistic Facial

Massage Bioflow Magnotherapy
Chinese Medicine
Homeopathy
Herbalism
Acupuncture
Soul Soothing
Gala-Now
Happy Days Holism
Holistic Touch
Thai Body and Foot Massage
Therapeutic Swedish
Inner Strength Treatments
Practical Natural Therapy
Deep Tissue Massage
Ayurvedic Massage
Therapeutic Massage
Pilates
Feng Shui
Shiatsu
Tai Chi
Palmist
Spiritual Advisor
Mentoring
Animal Aromatic (presumably only for animals)

At the same time as my original trawl for wares related to therapy was taking place, one of the city's two large bookstores was promoting the work of Geshe Kelsang Gyatso who writes about such topics as 'the Buddhist way to kindness and loving', and 'the clear light to bliss, tantric meditation, blissful journeys, and noble truths'. As part of the promotion, Gyatso was to give a talk on 'How to Solve Our Human Problems' during which 'peace of mind in these troubled times' would be offered. Unfortunately, I missed the presentation, and remain an angry trouble-maker.

But in this assessment of what is on offer to the consumer of anguish-relieving merchandise an advertisement placed in the newsagent's shop close to my house deserves a special mention:

Jay, Tarot Reader
Over 40 years experience reading Tarot.
Readings by appointment.

It was an unusual flier as this is not in an area of the city noted for fortune-tellers, psychics, mystics, telepaths, clairvoyants, or divinationists, although York itself does have its share of woozy winos, unfettered psychotics, ghost tours, and lost American (USA) tourists.

Tarot-reading is, in part, intended to assist with an individual's 'issue' (the catch-all phrase for whatever subject comes up during therapy). In that sense it resonates with other forms of mind exploration and remedy. In particular, using the Tarot appears to be 'life-coaching', with a bit of supernatural insight thrown in to ameliorate the customary terrestrial skills, qualities and knowledge of the therapist.

One British organization, Tarot UK, offers information about all things to do with this form of fortune-telling, a 'destiny-line' to get by telephone immediate predictions of impending events, and a possibly just a speedy mobile-phone texting service. 'Tarot-therapy' (which is my term, not that of Taro UK), is described thus:

> The Tarot is a powerful divination tool which can be used for making choices in life, but has historical associations with spirituality and the occult. Tarot readings can be used by clairvoyants and psychic seers as an oracle to assist you in choosing the life path which is best for you at any given crossroads in your life.
>
> (Tarot UK 2006)

A US-based organization, Tarot.com, provides an even clearer connection with a number of therapeutic approaches beyond that of spiritually-enhanced life-coaching:

> Transform your current life with a journey into past lives. Discover who you were, and how your past can influence your present and future.
>
> (Tarot.com 2006)

There is in essence, apart from the magic and a pack of pictographic playing cards, very little difference between, for example, psychodynamic therapy and this version of Tarot reading. Both require the client/customer to review his/her previous life in order to reconstruct the present and change prospective patterns of living.

The rules of life

I have never indulged in Tarot-reading, but I confess that I am a consumer of other psycho-soothing commodities (beyond therapy itself). Just before I got down to writing this book I bought Richard Templar's (2005) top-selling *The Rules of Life*. Another of my personal relationships had ended (or rather had stopped and re-commenced so many times that I couldn't decide what was going on). With the sub-title of 'A Personal Code for Living a Better, Happier, More Successful Kind of Life', this well-written book promised a lot.

While reading 'The Rules', as Templar refers to his 100 life-changing evocations, I was enthused greatly. The book pointed out concisely and clearly, and with boxed-one-line highlighted reminders, how to be a better person, how to make those around you love you, and how to make the world a better and more loving place in which to live. For about a week I smiled at strangers, was exceptionally nice to my then partner, thought before I acted, and had hope in my heart about all of humanity.

A week later, however, I had forgotten most of what Templar had taught me, and returned to my usual public persona (frowning regularly, frequently being obnoxious, and doing lots of things without any preparatory cerebral activity). Moreover, my incredulity about the human race had resurfaced with a vengeance. Of course it's not the product that is at fault but its owner. If only I had followed the specific rule in *The Rules of Life* that instructed the Rule Player (that's what Templar calls his acolytes) to practise habitually all of the other rules, then I'm sure I would have become near enough a perfect person (or at least much less grumpy and much more thoughtful).

But on the day (4th of June, 2006) that I set about revisiting Templar's handy summaries of each rule in a desperate last ditch attempt to feel better about me and be nicer to those with whom I come into contact, a lot of nasty events were happening in the wider world. An incident that especially drew a sharp contrast between goals of *The Rules* and real life concerned the scores of people reported as having been shot and killed execution-style in Iraq. Whilst I pampered myself with *The Rules*, the assassins' rules were cold-heartedly and barbarically ending the lives of children, youths, and adults.

The notion of *therapyitis* implies that global society becomes too engorged with therapy services and commodities; psychological distress may be alleviated, but relief is temporary and/or delusional; the underlying infection that produced the inflammation is not to be found in an individual's pathology, but in (global) society; the incessant pace of life; materialism; keeping up with technological advances; poverty; crime; *and* the incomprehensive banality of so-called popular entertainment (especially, day-time and reality television shows).

Emotional offsetting

Such 'emotional offsetting' (Tischner and Morrall 2007a) will never be effective. Emotional offsetting refers to the equivalent within therapy of 'carbon offsetting' within ecology. The practice of carbon offsetting provides absolution for those governments and corporations who seriously pollute the environment (through, for example, 'shock and awe' warfare, unregulated manufacturing processes, and cheap airplane travel). But, as George Monbiot (2007) points out, the planting of trees, erection of windmills, or attachment of methane-capturing equipment to the hindquarters of cows and pigs, does not deal effectively with the essential causes of global warming. Similarly, in therapy, the displacement of psychological distress through facile self-help programs and illusory professionalized helping, imparts absolution for those governments and corporations who seriously pollute the mind (through encouraging rampant consumerism, and not acting to stop inequalities and poverty), and does not deal with the essential causes of a malfunctioning global society.

Inflammation is the first response of the immune system to infection or irritation and may be referred to as the innate immune system and as 'healthy' nor 'unhealthy' on its own. Inflammation helps fight disease, but it comes at the cost of suspending the body's normal immune and catabolic processes. In the short term this is often a valid trade-off, but in the long term it causes progressive damage.

But far from therapy realizing its limitations in the way that Illich desired medicine to realize it, therapists are becoming more brazen in their claims to new territory. Psychoanalyst Darian Leader and science historian David Corfield (2007) argue that medical practice should be inundated with therapists. What they highlight is the irrefutable effect of the mind on the body, and presumably the reverse. Consequently, doctors should adopt psychosomatic medicine as their prime philosophical approach to treat diseases such as cancer, diabetes, and the common cold. Medical schools, they argue, should allow their students to study philosophy, and literature (and no doubt Freud) as much as science. Hence, Leader and Corfield consider therapy to be the senior partner in the budding medical-therapy alliance. Ironically, this also implies that therapyitis, far from being hazardous, is healthy for individuals and society.

It would seem that therapy is already so pervasive that it has attracted an unlikely convert. Rowan Williams, the Archbishop of Canterbury, in his 2004 Christmas address commented: 'He [God] is God so that he has the freedom to heal, to be our "therapist" ' (Williams 2004). Williams does not mention whether or not God is willing to undergo certification and registration.

Summary

Prior to God coming out as a therapist, Richard House (2003) recognized that therapy is more of spiritual practice than a profession. Less sympathetically than House, David Smail's (2006) view is that therapy is best described as 'medieval theology'. God, therefore, may feel at home within the therapeutic enterprise. Perhaps God, rather than remaining a simple minister of therapy, could be elevated to the status of divine guru for the *faith* of therapy. Certainly, if the 'opium of the people' (*Die Religion ... ist das Opium des Volkes*), as Karl Marx ([1843] 1970) described religion, was injected into therapy, it would exacerbate its infectiousness.

However, God's position on spreading therapy is somewhat conjectural. More prosaic alternatives to professionalization are that it should remain or become a craft (House 2003). The suggestion that therapy should be a 'craft' finds resonance in the work of Illich. Illich (in Illich et al. 1977) advocates the deprofessionalization and de-industrialization. Industrial society should, argues Illich, be replaced by a system of 'intermediate' technology. Technological production would be based on the needs of the community, rather than on the over-stimulated 'wants' created by the monolithic and alienating industrial conglomerates – and the professionals.

Virginia Ironside warns of the risks of professionalizing therapy:

> But I am extremely wary of therapists ever becoming in any way 'accredited'. Once you accredit them, encourage proper training, you are endorsing the idea that therapy is a valuable method of helping people, and one that works. And since I don't believe it does, to set up training schemes, and hand out diplomas, is about as useful as saying that quack doctors are only good if they are 'accredited quack doctors' ... They [therapists] may be genial people who do you no harm. They may well, with their warm smiles and interest in your well-being, give you healing comfort. But equally well, they may, actually, be exceptionally – and I mean exceptionally – dangerous.
>
> (Ironside 2006: 120–1)

There is a movement within the therapeutic enterprise that is hostile to the professionalized infectiousness of therapy. Set up in 1994, The Independent Practitioners Network (2006) is against the regulation and control. Rather than 'accreditation', members of the network propose self- and peer assessment. The network has 215 therapists associated with it, made up of 21 groups, with another 35 individuals looking for a group and a further dozen 'friends' (Independent Practitioners Network 2007).

However, although these few brave Independent Practitioners form a bastion of resistance against the certified hoards, they are likely to be overrun. Perhaps the 'war of manoeuvre', as Marxist and anti-fascist Antonio Gramsci in his famous 'Prison Notebooks' (1971) described a full-frontal attack on an opponent's power, is lost. What might be preferable is a 'war of position' using, for example, a propaganda campaign through which the failings of the therapeutic enterprise are publicized and the limits to therapy extolled. It may be wise first, however, to check which side can count on God.

CHAPTER 7

Insane

Certified
Psychiatry
Society

It was a memorable holiday, not least for confronting a colossal crocodile at close quarters, incestuous rhinos, fighting elephants, satiated lions, unknown (but very scary) wildlife in a rubbish dump at midnight, a precariously overloaded ferry (which a week later capsized, drowning 18 people), and me having to wear women's clothes (donated by Kirsty, my partner and travelling companion – mine having been left in another country by the airline). But this exploration of southern Africa was also outstanding because we had made a discovery as remarkable as David Livingstone had made in that region almost a century-and-half earlier.

Kirsty and I had spent a couple of weeks in Zambia staring at the Victoria Falls and at Australians from Victoria falling into them (while tied to a long elastic band), an hour illegally in Zimbabwe to get a better view of both, and a day in Namibia handing out boiled sweets to children. Respite was now needed from the inexorable vicissitudes that accompany the love of adventure ('wonder-of-the-world-boredom', bouncing Australians, border guards, and boiled sweets), and the adventure of love (Kirsty is a calm, considerate, giving and forgiving person, but borrowing her brand-new shorts and designer T-shirt had not gone down well).

We were now in the Botswana town of Kasane on the edge of Chobe National Park, and had seen more animals than have been photographed by National Geographic since its inception in 1888. Here we were to stumble across a social phenomenon that is as awesome to twenty-first-century explorers of the mind as finding the natural phenomenon of the *Mosi-oa-Tunya*[1] had been to nineteenth-century explorers of the land: a fail-proof, unpretentious, easy to use, method of measuring madness.[2] We named this vital psychometric tool the 'Botswana Mental Health Test'.[3]

During our stay in a lodge by the river Chobe, Kirsty and I were shown by our hosts, South Africans wishing to live in Botswana, 'Immigration Medical Form 4'. This form, a small part of the convoluted bureaucracy they had to undertake to gain residence in Botswana, was astonishing for its utter disregard of politically correct terminology and for its conceptual simplicity. Criterion used to assess the mental health status of the would-be immigrant could be considered crudely simplistic and staggeringly insensitive as well as tautological, teleological, and anomalous. Alternatively, they can be interpreted as refreshingly frank and penetratingly straightforward. They do cut-to-the-chase, call-a-spade-a-spade, and thereby undermine the propensity of the 'experts' in the mental health industry (psychiatrists, psychiatric nurses, and clinical psychologists) to obfuscate the obvious – in this case the obvious about madness.

The Republic of Botswana's Department of Immigration and Citizenship states that its objective is to facilitate legitimate residency, but also to protect cultural and economic stability by stopping entry by those it deems 'undesirable'. To assess the hazard 'undesirables' pose to Botswana, the Department of Immigration and Citizenship demands that applicants undergo medical examination. If you have one or more of a number of 'disabilities' it lists, you will not be allowed to reside in Botswana. Along with alcoholism and epilepsy, these disabilities include:

(a) Being an Idiot (a stupid person; imbecile; fool; a person of subnormal intelligence).

(b) Being an Imbecile (one whose mental development is above the level of idiocy but still below the norm).

(c) Being a Feeble-minded Person (weak in intellectual power; wanting firmness or constancy; irresolute; vacillating; imbecile).

(d) Having had a Previous Attack of Insanity ("A seriously impaired condition of the mental functions, involving the intellect, emotions, and will, or one or more of these faculties, exclusive of temporary states produced by and accompanying intoxications or acute febrile diseases.": *The Catholic Encyclopaedia*).

(e) Suffering from Constitutional Psychopathic Inferiority (The United States' 'Immigration Act, 1917' excluded from admission into the United States "persons of constitutional psychopathic inferiority" among others. Likewise, the Canadian 'Chinese Immigration Act, 1923' prohibited entry to Canada of Chinese immigrants who were deemed to be persons suffering "constitutional psychopathic inferiority").

(BBC 2002)

In a part of the world where medical services are in short supply, a pressurized examining doctor, wishing to speed up the assessment of the mental desirability of applicants, may need only to ask:

(a) Are you, or have you ever been, an idiot, imbecile, or feebleminded?
(b) Are you or have you ever been insane or a psychopath?

The second of these questions makes up the Botswana Mental Health Test, and equates to the usual cumulative and lengthy inquiries of psychiatric assessment. In the end, evaluation of mental fitness by a presiding practitioner or multidisciplinary team rests on the basic judgement 'is this person mad?'. Moreover, with only a tiny tweak to the test, the specific requirements of psychiatric post-liberal social control can also be satisfied. That is, by adding the rider 'And are you or have you ever been dangerous?' to the original question, the Botswana Mental Health Test can become the 'Botswana Mental Health and *Risk* Test'.

But of course the judgement about madness and dangerousness can only be considered to have been reached legitimately after the paraphernalia and opinions of the experts have been duly entertained. However, imagine two politically-correct would-be lovers who agonize over how to 'get it together' without seeming to be to the other presumptuous, sexist or exploitative. Eventually they are released from the agony of indecision when each realizes the other's already embedded raised consciousness about copulation. Then, with not much more than a 'nod-and-a-wink', they pursue their mutual desire. Ultimately, decisions about madness are made on nods-and-winks between those who have 'raised consciousness' about madness, and hence have the authority to make such pronouncements.

This is not, however, to ignore disagreements between experts. As with the two politically-correct lovers, tiffs do occur, their compelling lust tempered by disparities in their histories and from allegiances. Similarly, psychiatrists, psychiatric nurses, and clinical psychologists have divergences from their past and in their loyalties which interfere with what otherwise is their collective covetousness of madness.

Notwithstanding these internecine feuds, what unites the psychiatric disciplines of psychiatry, clinical psychology, and psychiatric nursing, is a medical conceptualization of madness. What is underplayed by the psychiatric disciplines is the social history and sociology of madness. Therapists, however, have little knowledge of *either* the medical or the social approaches to understanding madness.

Together with the ascriptions of dysfunctionality, arrogance, abusiveness, selfishness, and infectiousness (along with its deceitfulness, discussed in Chapter 8), the enterprise of therapy's ignorance *about* madness is as much an indication *of* madness as the 'neurotic' building a castle in the air and the 'psychotic' living in it. Therapy has both *constructed* and *occupied* its castles.

Consequently, I argue in this chapter that the therapeutic enterprise would fail the Botswana Mental Health Test and thereby be vulnerable to a diagnosis of insanity (if not idiocy). However, it as unethical for a sociologist to criticize therapy for the insane state of its enterprise and not provide pointers for change as it would be for a psychiatrist to blame the patient for his/her state of mind and withhold medication. The 'treatment' for therapy is to offer an injection of social historical and sociological insights into madness, thereby contributing further to its enlightenment.

Certified

To anthropomorphize either the abstract or the inanimate may seem an act of academic lunacy. However, there is precedent for regarding non-humans as having human qualities. Specifically, the sanity of social institutions and of society has previously been questioned.

Psychopathic corporations

Joel Bakan (2004) brands global corporations 'psychopathic'. Corporations can be so diagnosed, argues Bakan, because they are wantonly destructive.

They disregard the effect of their business operations on local settings, the lives of individuals, and the survival of humanity and the earth. Globalization has allowed large businesses to wreak environmental damage for profit, and destabilize the personal lives of workers by paying low wages, shedding jobs, and moving their operations if they find it financially expedient so to do or health and safety requirements become too stringent. Furthermore, the ethos of profit-making has caused a pandemic of materialism, commodification, and consumerism on terms dictated by big business:

> Over the last 150 years the corporation has risen from relative obscurity to become the world's dominant economic institution. Today, corporations govern our lives. They determine what we eat, what we watch, what we wear, where we work, and what we do. We are inescapably surrounded by their culture, iconography, and ideology.
>
> (Bakan 2004: 5)

Corporate power and its consequences are out of the control of governments and international organizations such as the United Nations. Rather, most governments have relented to the power of the corporation, and international organizations such as the World Bank and the International Monetary Fund, are vigorously supportive of globalized trade which *de facto* means corporate-controlled commerce.

Robert Hare (quoted in Bakan 2004) is an expert in psychopathy. He was invited by Bakan to assess the psychopathic nature of the corporation. Hare applied his checklist of psychological traits in humans, and determined that if corporations were human, they would be certified as psychopathic. Corporations, driven by profit, are unconcerned about the negative consequences of their business. They only become concerned about the damage they do to people and the planet when media, political, and public criticism threatens to undermine their market dominance. Concern expressed by corporations about these ill-effects (for example, in the form of 'social responsibility programmes') is superficial and manipulative:

> Human psychopaths are notorious for their ability to use charm as a mask to hide their dangerously self-obsessed personalities. For corporations, social responsibility may play the same role. Through it they can present themselves as compassionate and concerned about others when, in fact, they lack the ability to care about anyone or anything but themselves.
>
> (Hare, quoted in Bakan 2004: 56/57)

People, cultures, and even the planet are subjugated to corporate needs. At root, corporations as institutions are uncompromisingly selfish, observes Hare.

For Hare, however, the psychopathy of the corporation as an institution does not necessarily imply that its managers and chief executive are psychopaths. A few may be psychopaths, but most have families, friends, and some are extremely indulgent in their philanthropy to the benefit of humanity. Bill Gates, founder of the ubiquitous and omnipotent *Microsoft* corporation, has given US$ billions to charitable causes. Similarly, individual therapists, one supposes, are seldom psychopaths. Most also have families, friends, and are probably nice to their neighbours. It is the enterprise of therapy as a while, or organization subdivisions of it, that is 'constitutionally psychopathic'.

Insane society

Erich Fromm (1963) argues that it is all of (capitalist) society that is insane. Capitalism, for Fromm, is a type of social pathology akin to personal madness because it contains major contradictions and irrationalities. These symptoms of insanity, he claims, have immense social and economic consequences. For example, wars are fought regularly to defend markets and trade. Economic trading cycles produce periods of high unemployment and periods of worker shortage. Mass entertainment, promulgated purely for profit, 'dumbs down' human culture and human relations, thereby rendering life meaningless, and devoid of interpersonal intimacy.

However, Fromm, although prescient in his critique, did not predict the scale of humiliation for humanity that has been achieved in the twenty-first century. Much of what is broadcast on television, printed in the 'gutter' press and in popular magazines, released in films and DVDs, is promoted as 'sport' but dominated by corporate interests or those of wealthy oligarchs, and counts as 'information' or social discourse on the internet, is puerile in the extreme compared to what was available to the masses in the 1960s. Moreover, Fromm's criticism of capitalism's materialist ethic, whereby commodities are valued above everything else and hence displace spirituality and values based on people rather than inanimate objects, has become globalized.

Viviane Forrester has also pointed to the madness of the present economic system. The discrepancies in contemporary capitalism have, she argues, engendered what she describes as an 'economic horror'. She suggests that volatile employment conditions have become the norm, and that this has resulted in a type of 'social hell' for those who are marginalized:

Look for instance, at a luxurious, modern, sophisticated city, Paris, where so many people, the old or the new poor, sleep in the street, their bodies and minds wrecked by lack of nourishment, warmth, care, also togetherness and respect.

(Forrester 1999: 28)

Like Fromm, Forrester has been ahead of her time in envisaging the likely fall-out from these economic paradoxes. She realized that the rules of employment by the 1990s had become anachronistic. However, by the end of 2007 in her native France, the issue of employment rights (guaranteeing a certain level of pension and 'early' retirement) for millions of workers caused massive social disruption when the incoming president Nicolas Sarkozy decided to dismantle these rights (Sandford 2007). Can it be anything other than insanity to have one of the richest countries in the world, a world in which there are billions of people underemployed or unemployed, to elect a leader whose main task is to make that country richer by forcing those already in employment to work for more years, and, once retired from work, to receive less money to support their old age than has been agreed by their former leader? Are not these the economics of the madhouse?

Sociologist Iain Wilkinson (2005) postulates that there is a mass of data documenting social suffering in global society. What the data point to, for Wilkinson, is that the world is in turmoil with hundreds of millions of people brutalized through poverty, disease, and violence, or dehumanized through materialism. Furthermore, the meaning of the 'lived experiences' suffered by individuals is all but 'silenced' through the technocratic collection of this data and by the bureaucratic response. So, we (governments, corporations, people – you and me) *know* that global society has a split performance similar to the splintered emotions, thoughts, and behaviours of the psychotic. It is as if a psychiatrist is incomprehensively withholding from a clearly deranged patient suitable treatment.

Pathological ignorance

The madness of *therapy* is no better displayed than through its delusional (asocial) position on human suffering. But there is another massive misapprehension that therapy is guilty of, a paradox of gigantic proportions. Therapy has a myopic, misinformed, and misleading perception of the area of human performance that is integral to its enterprise – madness. Such an infirm grasp on the reality of its business is transparent derangement, and puts a different slant on the 'certification' of therapists.

Without madness, therapy would not exist. Madness inspired the enterprise that therapy has become. That is, it is Freud's recognition of what has become known as 'conversion disorder' (hysteria) kick-started psychotherapy. But therapists do not have adequate knowledge of the psychiatric basis of these subjects, let alone the sociology. It is psychiatry and sociology that have given the most informed, understandings of madness, given that there are disagreements between the two.

There is specialist therapy training and literature dedicated to various madnesses and for those in specific areas of practice. For example, cognitive-behavioural and emotional approaches for depression (Gilbert 2007), and mentalization-based treatment for borderline personality disorder (Bateman and Fonagy 2004). But, comprehensive information about madness, especially any sociological input, is conspicuous by its absence in basic therapy texts for therapists in non-specialist practice. Such knowledge should be standard.

For example, the *Handbook of Person-Centred Psychotherapy and Counselling* by Mike Cooper et al. (2007) has some information on madness, although this is mainly to do with schizophrenia. Fairing slightly better is Ray Woolfe et al.'s second edition of *Handbook of Counselling Psychology* (2003). Here there is a smidgen of madness as well as a dollop of sociology. Written by medical practitioners, *Medical and Psychiatric Issues for Counsellors* (Daines et al. 2007) contains, as would be expected, much medicalized madness but no reference to sociological considerations. What is common is the virtual absence of madness as is the case in Richard Nelson-Jones's fourth edition of the esteemed *Theory and Practice of Counselling and Therapy* (2005), and Val Wosket's *Egan's Skilled Helper Model* (2006).

Hence, in the main, therapy is neither in its theoretical formulations nor in its practice applications, operating from a suitably informed basis. This is both unscholarly and immoral. Moreover, such ignorance means therapy is ineffectual.

Mad as each other

During Heather's formal therapy sessions (accepting that she only had a handful, and that she had more than one therapist), little headway was made in revealing, let alone comprehending the range and roots of her psychological distress. Therefore, the possibility that she was suffering from madness was not investigated suitably. Len's view came to be, although by then his opinion was decidedly tainted by their troubled interactions, sex, and love, that Heather was not medically mad. Her performance did skirt the edges of diagnosable anxiety, depression, hypomania, obsessional-compulsive disorder, intermittent explosive disorder, and especially troublesome-personality-changes disorder.[4] But these displays *de la folie* were remarkably well contained. Heather, Len guessed, was unendingly troublesome to Heather, but only infrequently, albeit very dramatically, to others. Heather's 'moods so foul' (Len's Cohenesque description of her temperament as Mr Hyde rather than Dr Jekyll), were vented on selected intimates and strangers. Heather was for the most part able to present the illusion of being what Erving Goffman (1963) described as one of the 'normals'.

What Heather does suffer from, Len believed, is an undocumented syndrome. This was the combination of the documented syndromes of '*idiot savant*' and '*genius savant*'. That is, Heather's outstanding capacity for incisive reasoning, erudite diction, electrifying exuberance, virtuoso musical accomplishments, photographic memory, inspired drollness, and perfectionist impulse, coincides with obtuse stubbornness, maladroit moodiness, and absurd assumptions.

To be fair, Heather didn't believe that Len was a normal. A prevailing theme in their interchanges was the question of which one of them was really the mad one. With the romantic sensitivity of mating wildebeests, Len responded to Heather's many entreaties for them to marry with the condition that she first satisfy the demands of the Botswana Mental Health Test. It was testament to his feelings for her that he offered to help her revise for the examination (as he had done with her academic studies), and gave her anti-madness self-help literature as presents (wisely, always accompanied by such emotional emollients as red wine or cocoa-rich chocolate). But Len was to concede that by the terminal stage of their crazy relationship, which until then had only caused him insomnia, he had indeed succumbed to insanity.

Therapy is a mad business

Claiming that therapists are ignorant about their trade may seem unduly harsh. Ignorance of sociology may be excusable especially if rectified. Moreover, such subjects as neuro-biology and neuro-psychology, genetics, and evolutionary psychology, are as imperative to the education of sociologists as they should be to therapists. In this age of technological and scientific revolution, global mass electronic communications, and hyper-information, disciplinary tribalism based on discrete knowledge is inappropriate. Dismantling the knowledge boundaries of *all* disciplinary tribes is paramount for global society to progress beyond its present messy state.

But the ignorance of therapy about madness is indefensible.

Psychological distress is what brings most, if not all, clients to want to have therapy. It is hard to imagine what else an individual would want with therapy. There are of course 'therapy addicts' who misuse the service of therapists, or are misused in the service of therapists. Some people may stumble into therapy not realizing what it is, possibly sent by their general practitioner because of a difficulty in making a diagnosis and a homeopath or acupuncturist is unavailable. Perhaps others have been bought a therapy session as a 'gift' for their birthday, or simply wishes to experience for themselves what their friends are doing. There is no reason why in a world where there is a 'commodification of everything' therapy cannot become akin to the one-off 'balloon ride' or 'bungee jump', or be another 'one more thing to do before I die' along with visiting the Taj Mahal, the Grand Canyon, and a lap-dance club.

However, apart from the habituated, those with idiopathic illness, thrill-seekers, and inveterate consumers, the remaining client population attend therapy because their minds are in a mess. They are mad.

But describing the genuine customers of the therapeutic enterprise as mad does depend on how madness is conceptualized. It also depends on how much adherence there is to a particular tribal discourse. Some of these tribal discourses either deny that madness exists at all, mangle the English language to produce dishonest, obfuscated, oxymoronic, and euphemistic phrases such as: 'mental health services' (services are for mental disorder not mental health); 'mental health practitioners' (nurses and doctors, and the allied disciplines deal with the mental disordered not the mentally healthy); 'mental health problems' (such problems are symptoms of a mental disorder, rather than as this sloppy slogan implies, difficulties with being mentally healthy); 'mental health disorders' (this expression is too ridiculous to bother deciphering); and 'psychiatrically challenged' (a mixture of medicalization of the mad and political-correctness gone mad: but at least it has the merit of encouraging a wry smile from those to whom it is conveyed).

The therapist refers to the client's 'issues' or (in the case of Heather) 'troubles', the psychiatrist to the patient's 'illness' or 'disorder', and the clinical psychologist may utilize both therapeutic and medical terminology. But it is only a matter of selective discourse-based interpretation that distinguishes 'loss-reaction' from 'clinical depression', stress from 'anxiety state', or existential-phenomenological episode from schizophrenia.

Sociologists (along with social historians and anthropologists) see these issues and troubles, and illnesses and disorders, as a type of social deviance – madness.

Madness is therefore what therapy is about. That is, historical and contemporary therapies are either designed explicitly or implicitly to mine, manufacture, manage, or masque madness. Moreover, the issue a client discusses with a therapist and the mental health illness a patient is diagnosed with by his/her general practitioner could be considered essentially indistinguishable. That is, it is a matter of providence, availability of specialist services, and personal choice, finances and social capital, as to whether or not an individual becomes subsumed under therapy or psychiatry. The exceptions would be some of those people who are intensely mad, those who want but cannot pay for private therapy, do not know how to engage in the process of obtaining a counsellor or do not have the required skills and attitudes of being a client (for example, wanting to change their lives, and being able to communicate effectively enough to participate in therapy).[5]

Psychiatry

There certainly seems to be a lot of madness around in the world, and apparently more on its way. Social historian Roy Porter (2003) suggests that today's society is suffering from 'mental hypochondria'. The World Health Organization (WHO) envisages that mental disorder will soon be one of, if not *the*, most serious global health problem:

- Hundreds of millions of people worldwide are affected by mental, neurological or behavioural problems at any time.
- 877,000 people die by suicide every year.
- Mental illnesses are common to all countries and cause immense suffering.
- One in four patients visiting a health service has at least one mental, neurological or behavioural disorder, but most of these disorders are neither diagnosed nor treated.
- Mental illnesses affect and are affected by chronic conditions such as cancer, heart and cardiovascular diseases, diabetes and HIV/AIDS. Untreated, they bring about unhealthy behaviour, non-compliance with prescribed medical regimens, diminished immune functioning, and poor prognosis.
- Cost-effective treatments exist for most disorders and, if correctly

applied, could enable most of those affected to become functioning members of society.

- Barriers to effective treatment of mental illness include lack of recognition of the seriousness of mental illness and lack of understanding about the benefits of services. Policy makers, insurance companies, health and labour policies, and the public at large – all discriminate between physical and mental problems.
- Most middle and low-income countries devote less than 1% of their health expenditure to mental health. Consequently mental health policies, legislation, community care facilities, and treatments for people with mental illness are not given the priority they deserve.

(WHO 2008)

Medicalized madness

The ascendant explanation of madness has emerged from Western medicine, and is spreading globally. Madness is construed as 'disorder' or 'illness' akin to physical ailments. Specialist medical practitioners (psychiatrists) take the lead in defining and resolving madness. Medicine portrays a world without psychiatry as one of mysticism, cruelty, and devoid of effective treatment and genuine compassion (Shorter 1997). Medicine is not blind to its failures (such as the wacky management of the madness of King George III, and the futile spinning and dousing so popular in the nineteenth-century madhouse). But the version of the history of madness favoured by medicine is characterized by improved understandings of causation, treatments that work, and humane care (Johnstone 2000).

The medical profession collaborates with national government health departments and international health organizations in the formulation and distribution of facts and figures about, and classifications of, psychological distress. There are two main classification systems. The first, the International Classification of Diseases (ICD–10), is compiled by WHO. The second is the Diagnostic and Statistical Manual of Mental Disorders of the American Psychiatric Association (DSM–IV).

However, the fact that there *are* two systems of classification, and that both regularly revise their contents, suggests that psychiatric diagnosis is not constant and universal. Aspects of human performance deemed indicative of mental disorder or normality today may not have been so categorized yesterday or might not be tomorrow. Moreover the classification indexes have thousands of categories and sub-categories of disorder including: numerous types of schizophrenia, depression, mania, anxiety, compulsions and obsessions, personality disorder, delirium, psychosomatic syndromes, dementia, and eating difficulties with body weight. Also included are stuttering, stealing, frotteurism, voyeurism, fetishism, female orgasmic disorder, and male hypoactive-sexual-desire disorder.

Such a wide-ranging conceptualization of disorder overlaps with understandings of normality to the point of rendering some so-called psychiatric conditions meaningless. Furthermore, madness may be considered an understandable reaction to mad circumstances (Laing 1965; Laing and Esterson 1964), a point on a scale of human performance that does not partition ordinariness from oddness (Bentall 2003), or a way of being that should be celebrated (Dellar et al. 2000).

Every society separates some of its 'deviants' from the 'normals' on the basis of a perceived 'difference' which does not seem to fit other categories of deviant human performance (such as criminality, drunkenness, impoverishment, religiosity, and 'New Age' lifestyles). There is a discernible 'strangeness' which is disturbing in the performance of certain individuals. Whether it is called 'Amok' (Malaysia), 'Pibloktoq' (the Arctic), 'Bena Bena' (New Guinea), 'Imu' (Japan), 'Koro' (China), 'Windigo' (native North Americans), or witchcraft (medieval Europe), the social deviance of 'strangeness' is acknowledged and set apart from normality. Setting apart may mean either social distancing or social control (with possible physical segregation). In the West, politically astute manoeuvring by medicine has resulted in the medicalization of this strangeness and psychiatrists becoming the arbiters of segregation.

The medicalization of madness, however began thousands of years ago. Porter (1987; 2003) explains that the antecedents of medicalized madness in the West can be traced to the holistic explanatory schema for health and disease of Ancient Greece and Rome. For Hippocrates and Galen, physical and mental health and disease were interlinked. Humoral theory in particular (levels of black bile, yellow bile, phlegm, and blood needed to be in balance with each other to maintain good health), made both the body and the mind the province of medical practitioners.

Although religious and folk beliefs prevailed, Porter records that Islamic and Christian medicine in medieval times continued this interest in the association of the mind with the body. Melancholia and mania were popular diagnostic categories.

Segregation, although home-based, also came along early, as did the perception that seriously disturbed people could be dangerous. Plato advised that 'if a man is mad' (presumably this also applied to mad women), his family must not let him roam in the city to prevent injury to himself, to others, and to property (Porter 2003). While those kept at home might be tethered, kept in a pen or cellar, those perceived as harmless did roam towns and countryside during and after the ancient civilizations living by begging (Shorter 1997).

Incarceration

Institutional segregation began in England in the thirteenth century when the St Mary of Bethlehem of London ('Bedlam'), a religious order providing care for the physically sick, began to accept the mad. Other institutions were set up in continental Europe by the beginning of the Renaissance in the fifteenth century. In the seventeenth century around 6,000 mad people were incarcerated in the *Hôpital Général de Paris*, and incarceration of the mad was then to spread throughout France (Porter 2003). Michel Foucault in his seminal work on madness *Histoire de la folie à l'âge classique* (1961) asserts that this is the age of the 'great confinement', and that the mad were henceforth debased to the degree of being rendered little more than wild beasts. There was, suggests Foucault, a 'great conspiracy' by governments and the propertied classes to separate reason from unreason. Industrialization and capitalist economics required rationality together with order and diligence. Irrational undesirables (the mad) had to be removed from the gaze of the public. Segregated social control of madness began on a massive scale.

However, Porter challenges Foucault's proposition, arguing that apart from France, there was no 'great confinement' of the mad in Europe at this time. For example, it was not until the middle of the nineteenth century that the majority of asylums were built to confine the mad in England. Moreover, the planning of institutional confinement was not centralized, but organized locally. Furthermore, although the madness business was profitable to the private owners of madhouses, frequently the institutions were built for philanthropic and humanitarian ideals and not simply to benefit those wishing to inculcate rationalism in society.

What institutional segregation undoubtedly did provide was a captive audience on whom doctors could experiment and thereby develop their sub-speciality of psychiatry. Taking England as an exemplar, the asylums had not been built for the medical profession, but doctors were, as local notables, invited to oversee their administration. This they did relatively well, given the conditions the mad would otherwise have had to live under with their families or roaming the land. Medical experimentation started with physical restraint, cold baths, hot baths, rotating mechanism, blood-letting, purges, and emetics, and eventually led to electro-convulsant therapy, psycho-tropic drugs, and psycho-surgery.

Asylums were forbidding and oppressive places in which to be committed perhaps for years if not life. Inmates were habitually mistreated by their keepers, and sometimes their doctors. But this had not been the intention behind such massive financial investment in housing the mad. However, institutions which sponsored 'moral treatment', supported by lay bene-factors and religious groups, emerged in France, England, Italy, and the USA late in the eighteenth century and continued throughout the nineteenth century as alternatives to the asylums based on physical treatments (and episodic cruelty).

But the medical control of madness was not to be thwarted. Employing a technique for occupational advancement which has served the profession of medicine extraordinarily well, moral treatment was to be incorporated into mainstream psychiatric care. The profession of medicine had by the end of the nineteenth century monopolized the market in madness. Psychiatry was well established as a medical area of expertise, and madness had become as much an 'illness' or 'disorder' as lung disease or liver failure.

Decarceration

A new age of community care arrived in the early part of the twentieth century in Europe and the USA. This movement to de-institutionalize the mad was assisted by the discovery of chemicals in France and the USA that could dampen down psychotic symptoms. The discovery of these drugs, the financial difficulties of continuing to operate huge institutions, and a change in Western culture towards more tolerance and liberty of such undesirables, meant widespread decarceration (Miller and Rose 1986; Scull 1984).

Losing its power-base (what had become the mental hospital) did affect the dominance of psychiatry. The anti-psychiatry movement, social work, psychology, therapy, and the uppity discipline of psychiatric nursing had dented the dominance of medicine. However, the power of psychiatry, and therefore the medicalization of madness, have since been boosted con-siderably by the arrival of new psycho-pharmacological products, the development of sophisticated diagnostic technology, improvements in psycho-surgery, and the accomplishment of the genome map.

Society

The social history of psychiatry aside, there are specific sociological reflections that either complement or contradict the medical view on madness. What is common to all sociological thought is that the effect of society on the manufacture and maintenance of madness is substantial.

Structural madness

Structuralist sociologists in essence accept medical notions of disease. What they argue is that, although there are actual diseases, the effect of society on health should be seen to be the greatest determinant of good and bad health. Professor William Cockerham from the University of Alabama, USA, makes the point well:

> [T]he social context can shape the risk of exposure, the susceptibility of the host, and the disease's course and outcome – regardless of whether the disease is infectious, genetic, metabolic, malignant, or degenerative ... This includes major afflictions like heart disease, Type 2 diabetes, stroke, cancers like lung and cervical neoplasms, HIV/AIDS and other sexually-transmitted infections, pulmonary diseases, kidney disease and many other ailments.
>
> (Cockerham 2005: 1–2)

One of these 'other ailments' is madness.

Specifically, the stucturalist argues that the position an individual holds within a social hierarchy which is differentiated by wealth correlates directly with disease and mortality. Global society is so structured. The further down the hierarchy a person is positioned, the more chronic illnesses he/she will suffer, and the earlier in life he/she will die. Moreover, people on the bottom of the social hierarchy suffer from madness far more than those at the top. For example, there is a strong connection between (lower) social groups, and alcohol and drug addiction, schizophrenia, depression, Alzheimer's disease, and personality disorder. A number of types of madness, however, occur more frequently among those further up the hierarchy. Theses are eating disorders, manic-depression (bipolar disorder), and anxiety (Cockerham 2005). The structuralist also acknowledges that gender, ethnicity, and geography play a part in the generation of infirmity and maintenance of well-being.

A structuralist position is taken by Andrew Scull (1979; 1984; 1992). He refers to the function of psychiatry as an agency of social control. The mad, for Scull, are socially positioned within the proletariat. Psychiatry directly serves the capitalist state by controlling the mad. For Scull, the shift from incarceration to community care was purely an economic decision and had little to do with the discovery of new drugs or progressive ideas. However, drugs (and therapy) have become the way to manage madness in the community. The ghettoization and impoverishment of the mad after decarceration predicted by Scull have materialized. Community as the only policy for the mad has become discredited in countries such as Britain,

Australia, and the USA, and more institutional segregation is being rein-troduced especially for those deemed dangerous (Morrall and Hazelton 2004; Hazelton and Morrall 2008).

A variety of the structuralist approach is taken by social disorganization theorists. From this perspective, the (dis)organization of urban areas causes madness along with criminality. As far back as the 1960s, Robert Faris and Warren Dunham (1965) were suggesting that the design of cities had an important effect on human performance. Most of global society is now either living in cities or drifting towards them. While their knowledge of mid-nineteenth-century cities doesn't necessarily apply accurately to twenty-first-century metropolitan conurbations, they have provided interesting observa-tions about the social causation of deviance. Their argument was that cities can be broken down into a number of 'concentric-zones'. The specific characteristics of each zone either enhanced, reduced or increased deviancy. At the centre of the city was the zone that contained the commercial sector, containing shops, offices, small factories, and places of entertainment. The mentally disordered are represented disproportionately in this zone, which also serves as the sleeping and begging arena for the homeless and supplies opportunities for a large amount of petty criminal activity.

The zone surrounding this innermost area is typified by slum housing, ghettos, and rented accommodation. Here reside new immigrants, the lower working class (semi-skilled and unskilled workers, many of whom are only partially employed), the 'underclass' (the permanently unemployed, drug users and dealers, and prostitutes), and students. If and when the members of these groups move up the social hierarchy they have the opportunity to enter the third zone, which accommodates the 'stable working class' as well as former immigrants who are now more established within the social system. In the case of students, when their studies are completed, they may move away altogether and further up the social hierarchy.

In many Western countries, segments of these three zones have been 'gentrified'. That is, certain sections of the middle class (who are usually relatively young, either single or cohabiting, and without children) have either begun living in previously dilapidated housing which have been 'converted' or are renting a fashionable apartment. Closeness to the city centre offers childless, young employed people with a large amount of disposable income, easy access to their work and entertainment.

Situated on the edge of the city in the last of Faris and Dunham's zones the residential suburbs are to be found. These have traditionally been inhabited by the middle class, but there is a growing trend certainly in Britain for some of this group reside in the countryside and travel into the city for work.

It is not the personal performance of the people attached to these zones that creates their distinguishing features, argue Faris and Dunham. Rather it is the physical environment that dictates how people perform (either as normals or deviants). Each zone keeps its identity despite the movement of groups through its parameters. But, where there is significant population movement, the anonymity and social isolation that this movement produces, mean that crime and madness will flourish.

Moreover, Robert Merton (1938), utilizing Emile Durkheim's concept of 'anomie', argued that communities and societies that were 'strained' because of factors such as a rapid population turnover, warfare, or economically and political failure, could induce debilitation in individuals. What these people experience is aimlessness, insecurity, and despair that could lead to suicide.

Mad labels and mythical madness

Labelling theory, derived from interactionist sociology, is an approach that does not accept madness as real in the medical sense. Labelling theorist Thomas Scheff's (1966) proposition is that mental disorder is 'residual' rule-breaking. That is, when all other categories of deviance have been exhausted, then the label of 'madness' will be applied by the agencies of social control (for example, the police and judiciary), and authenticated by psychiatry. Scheff also pointed out that this deviancy label of last resort was likely to have permanent negative consequences for individual, shaping both his/her self-identity and the perception of others towards him/her. For Goffman (1963), the individual so labelled became stigmatized, socially discredited, ending up with what he called a 'spoiled identity'. The spoiled identity of the mad, however, had been long while in the making, according to Foucault, but ending with the undignified label of beast due to their perceived 'unreason' when reason was the order the things.

Thomas Szasz goes further than Scheff and argues that madness is a myth, and therefore the practice of psychiatry is illusory. Moreover, similar to Ivan Illich's view of all of the medical profession, Szasz claims that psychiatry disables rather than enables its patients. By classifying everyday obstacles as illness or disorder, people do not deal with their lives effectively:

> It is customary to define psychiatry as a medical speciality concerned with the study, diagnosis, and treatment of mental illnesses. This is a worthless and misleading definition. Mental illness is a myth. Psychiatrists are not concerned with mental illnesses and their treatments. In actual practice they deal with personal, social, and ethical problems in living.
>
> (Szasz 1972: 269)

For Szasz, 'problems in living' are not the province of medical science. Medical science should only deal with conditions that have identifiable organic origin. The origin of, for example, schizophrenia, may be found to be genetic. Other diseases listed in the DSM and ICD do have known biological causation. But most of madness still cannot be linked to organic dysfunction.

Szasz accuses psychiatry of projecting a falsely correlating 'diagnosis' with 'disease'. Diagnoses are fabricated epithets attributed to 'symptoms' (usually behaviours) which may or may not have links to actual disease. There is, points out Szasz, obvious compatibility between the diagnostic designation of 'malaria' and pathological bodily changes. There is, he postulates, no such synchronicity between psychiatric symptoms such as believing in devils, feeling despondent, or restless, and the 'illnesses' they purport to represent (schizophrenia, depression, and an anxiety state). This, argues Szasz, is why some psychiatric ailments (for example, masturbatory insanity, and homosexuality) disappear from psychiatric taxonomies. Mental diseases, states Szasz (1993), have only the status of metaphor and should not be taken literally.

Szasz illustrates the fallibility of psychiatric diagnostic systems by exposing how they are constructed. He observes that the formal classification systems come about through a consensus being reached by a panel of psychiatric experts who make or break particular human performances as a disease. That is, it is opinion rather than empirical observation of pathology that counts.

The mentally disordered, argues Szasz, have been demonized, segregated, and mistreated because the state *does* distinguish between being sick from pathogens and madness. Psychiatry is actually performing as an agency of social control far more than as a genuine medical speciality. What Szasz (1972) advocates is the liberalization of society along free-market principles. The state and psychiatry should be stripped of their powers with respect to madness. Psychiatry should leave misery, agitation, and bad and excessive behaviours to other non-medical disciplines. That is, people, who have problems in living (and that would be most of the world's population in one way or another), should hire lawyers or *therapists*!

Summary

Thomas Szasz has a lot to offer the enterprise of therapy. First, he provides an argument for the therapeutic enterprise to dismiss the tag I have placed at its door of insanity. He doesn't believe that individuals suffer from insanity because there is no such medical phenomenon. If he is correct, then it is hardly logical to claim that a social institution can be so described. Second, although he is adamant that psychiatry should not be in the business of helping people with their life problems, other disciplines should. What's more, these other disciplines should earn money from such help. Given the amount of help that's likely to be required for the millions if not billions of people in global society with 'problems in living', this is very good news for those occupations he regards as in the frontline of problem solving – lawyers and therapists.

However, there are caveats to this good news. First, Szasz's acceptance that organic pathology must be the mainstay of medical work, if applied to therapy, may reinstate its insane certification. It is not pathology in individual therapists that is the concern here (apart from a few), but the *organic* pathology of the enterprise of therapy. By organic pathology I am referring to the dysfunctional bureaucratic and ideological workings of the therapeutic enterprise.

Second, Szasz is quite simply wrong. Madness is 'real' in the sociological realist sense. No matter what the cultural connotations to its formulation, no matter whether measured by objective science or by subjective phenomenological experience, real people suffer from real symptoms of psychological distress and want real relief from them. Moreover, there are demonstrable physical alterations to bodily function that may be either cause or effect, but are not merely metaphorical. Contemporary psychiatry has tools to show how the mind affects the body and vice versa. Although it has not perfected its treatments, some physical treatments, while not offering necessarily a cure, do allow mad people to live sane lives. While social power, labelling, and stigma impinge on human performance, the psychiatric and structural sociological positions have a far more realistic appraisal of madness.

So the bottom line for me is, if I or one of my friends/relatives were succumb to madness, it is the services of a psychiatrist (with a good reputation) that may be called upon. It most definitely is *not* a deconstructionist sociologist or anti-psychiatrist (regardless of their reputations). Furthermore, I have used and would certainly use again and suggest to others, the services of therapists but only those who have a good reputation, are informed about madness, *and* are capable of passing the Botswana Mental Health Test.

CHAPTER 8

Deceitful

Nirvana

Shangri-La

Reality

As psychologist John Schumaker (2006) observes, people in Western society are being conned into becoming mental-masturbatory 'happichondriacs'. The foundations of the deception are both scientifically and philosophically shaky. Theories and techniques to transcend barriers to blissfulness have come to pass from experiments with anal insertions, unfolding the life-extending habits of the pious, questioning why slum-dwellers in Calcutta are more contented than they should be, and comparing highly complex global society with an anachronistic medieval kingdom where women and men have to wear dresses (admittedly, of different lengths).

All Heather ever wanted to be, she told Len, was happy. This platform for leading her life, Heather explained, had been handed to her and her brother by their mother who, for the best of motives, wanted her children 'just to be happy'. Heather's mother, however, although not intentionally hypocritical, had said one thing but done another. With considerable emotional cost, she had carved out a career against the cultural norms of her upbringing and her husband's idea of the role of a wife. But, in an unusually candid moment of contemplation and intimacy, Heather confessed to Len that it had come as quite a shock to find at the age of 40 that happiness wasn't all it was cracked up to be. Just 'being happy' might stem from, but didn't lead to, an interesting job, a fulfilling relationship, owning a house with a big garden, and having a plentiful pension. Although unstated by Heather, Len assumed that the absence of these attainments had severely exacerbated Heather's feelings of insecurity and rejection.

Heather has some illustrious bedfellows in questioning the rationale for the pursuit of happiness. The nineteenth-century British utilitarian philosopher and Member of Parliament John Stuart Mill suggested that dissatisfaction was a higher human quality than satisfaction. Human beings have faculties more elevated than the needs of animals, and, when once made conscious of them, cannot find and sustain happiness if these superior needs are not gratified. Humans should endeavour to use their intellect and morality in the struggle to understand and change the world. Only when their superior consciousness and conscience were utilized effectively would they achieve happiness: 'Human beings have faculties more elevated than the animal appetites and, when once made conscious of them, do not regard anything as happiness which does not include their gratification' (Mill [1861] 2001: 8). Mill linked individual happiness to a happy society. That is, unhappy humans would use their intellect and morality to make decisions which would furnish a fair and just social system. For Mill, only animals or human dunces and ignoramuses are happy with the satisfaction of base pleasures:

> It is better to be a human being dissatisfied than a pig satisfied; better to be Socrates dissatisfied than a fool satisfied. And if the fool, or the pig, are of a different opinion, it is because they only know their own side of the question. The other party to the comparison knows both sides.
>
> (Mill [1861] 2001: 10)

Consequently, Mill postulated that those humans with the very highest intellect and moral standing suffered the most. Moreover, once consciousness and conscience are raised, there is no turning back. Those of superior thinking and ethical standards cannot any more gain contentment from only relieving their primary needs (hunger, food, shelter, and sex), an undemanding occupation, or, what Eric Fromm (1963) refers to as 'dumb' popular entertainment.

So, with global society in the mess it is today, those people deemed to be happy are really ill-informed or idiots, or both. However, the 'great deceit' being promulgated about achieving happiness is founded on the simplistic notion that those who report being happy occupy the cultural *high ground* towards which all global citizens should travel, not the intellectual and moral *low ground* above which humanity should transcend.

Happiness has a long history (although so does suffering, much favoured as the ideal human condition by one or two of the main religions). It has inspired philosophical entreaties as far back as Ancient Graeco-Roman civilization (particularly Aristotle and Epicurus), as being an important consideration for the Enlightenment theorists. Happiness has also been politicized. For example, the achievement of happiness is an absolute right enshrined in the USA Declaration of Independence (Bond 2003).

But happiness has now become huge. There is a profitable and expanding industry selling messages and methods designed to erase glumness from the world, or at least from those who can afford to buy their way into joy-fulness. The study of happiness has generated university courses throughout the Western world, senior academic posts, journals, and empirical research. A private school in England has added happiness to the 'personal, social and health education' part of its curriculum for 14–16 year olds (Ward 2006). Journalist Oliver Burkeman (2006) notes that the internet retailer Amazon listed about 20,000 self-help books in 2001, but by 2006 this had risen to over 61,000. A year later when I checked Amazon's listings, the figure for self-help books was nearly 85,000 (and 1,763 DVDs).

Feeding the commercialization of happiness is the 'positive' strand of psychology (Snyder and Lopez 2004). That is, positive psychology is helping to commodify an emotional state.

Positive psychology originated in the USA. Martin Seligman, Professor of Psychology at the University of Pennsylvania is the foremost authority of the 'positive' division of psychology. Seligman, having invented positive psychology, has developed a programme to assess and improve an indivi-dual's happiness quotient (Seligman 2007). The programme is accessible on the website of the 'Happiness Center'. So effusively positive is the pro-gramme's promotional blurb about the ease of the psychological voyage to nirvana that a 90 per cent success rate is promised. However, classic marketing strategies are also used (freebies) to further entice consumers:

We are so confident that this program will help you, we've developed a no-obligation, limited-time offer to try Dr. Seligman's powerful pro-gram for one month free. This free offer includes the first Happiness Building Exercise that has helped so many of our members fight

depression in as little as 15 days! If after your first month, you feel the
Reflective Happiness Program hasn't helped, you'll owe nothing.

(Happiness Center 2007)

Nick Baylis is Co-Director of the Well-being Institute, University of Cambridge, and Fellow of the Royal Society of Arts for the Encouragement of Arts, Manufacture and Commerce. 'Dr Nick' is both effusively positive and expansive. Baylis states that his 'lessons' can be applied to individuals, their communities and societies:

Welcome! I'm Dr Nick Baylis.

Based at Cambridge University since 1994, I'm a Well-being Scientist and Practising Psychologist attempting to understand the hows and whys of wonderful lives, looking for the most promising routes to healthy, helpful, and good-hearted living.

In my first ever book, *Learning from Wonderful Lives: Lessons from the Study of Well-being*, I explain what we've discovered so far. I have written this for a very general readership so that everyone can benefit from all the principles and strategies, skills and experiences, that seem to help life go better, no matter where we're starting from.

This new Institute promotes the scientific study of well-being.

Well-being studies can focus at the level of an individual or partnership, a family or organization, or a community and wider society. The knowledge they generate can be applied to foster lives that are healthy psychologically, socially and physically, and working in harmony with the natural environment.

(Baylis 2006)

This 'Dr Nick' should not be confused with the (fictional) effusively expansive 'Dr Nick' from *The Simpsons* cartoon television series, a likeable and amusing but grandiose and dubious medical practitioner. The cartoon Dr Nick did, however, receive a glowing tribute as a modern doctor keeping his patients happy by trying to meet their every whim by (real) physicians in the Canadian Medical Association Journal (Patterson and Weijer 1998).

Such effusively positive expansiveness is replicated by another positive psychologist, Tal Ben-Shahar. Indeed, Ben-Shahar appears to have global domination in mind for positive psychology. Ben-Shahar is a lecturer in the School of Positive Psychology at Harvard University. Apparently, his course in positive psychology attracts more students than any other at Harvard. In his self-help book *Happier: Finding Pleasure, Meaning and Life's Ultimate Currency* (2007) Ben-Shahar utilizes the 'science' of positive psychology to argue that anyone can learn to be happy (or at least happier). On his website he describes himself 'as an avid sportsman', refers to his consultative role in advising corporate executives, the public, and what he describes as 'at risk groups'. To the left of a picture of himself on a sofa dressed casually but looking thoughtful if slightly pensive, and above another picture of him dressed more formally but definitely looking happier, are these words in large type:

Tal Ben-Shahar
Teaching the World to Focus on the Good

Ben-Shahar like Seligman, knows something about selling. However, rather than a free month's trial, Ben-Shahar gives away 'happiness tips' (six of them). Interestingly if not somewhat disconcerting, ten minutes after I had first entered Ben-Shahar's website another picture appeared replacing the one of him wearing a collar and tie. This time both of the pictures showed him dressed casually. The replacement, however, had him carrying about ten books. Despite some of the books appearing to be rather bulky, his smile and positive outlook stayed. I don't imagine that Ben-Shahar is live on 'webcam' altering his style of dress repeatedly to tempt possible happiness consumers in a similar way to those trying to sell sex commodities on the internet (accepting that they are much more likely to be taking their clothes off rather than replacing them). But the sales technique is much the same.

I am sceptical about the hard-nose corporate executives and career academics who ply this trade in happiness being totally indoctrinated by their own enthusiastic sales pitches. Like any other merchandise, their advertisements may not live up to the actuality. Commercials for cars commonly show impeccable people having improbable driving experiences whereby winding empty roads through glorious countryside or channels materialize through otherwise gridlocked cities as soon as the driver turns the ignition key. So, promises of happiness have to be marketed in an idealistic form. The publishers and maharishis of positiveness could hardly be openly lukewarm or equivocal about their product, just as the car manufacturers and sales staff are unlikely to point that their vehicles will be driven by imperfect people probably queuing in lines of traffic for much of the time.

Therapists are collaborators in the business of bliss. But, unlike their more astute entrepreneurial and academic co-conspirators (who face constant and intense commercial and research pressures to promote happiness), they are both deluding and deluded. That is, not only do therapists propagate the myth of merriness, but they have succumbed to self-indoctrination. They are disciples *and* evangelists. It is as if the lunatics have not only taken over the asylum, but so convinced are they that it is the rest of the world which is mad and not themselves, they have formed community 'out-reach' teams to provide treatment (compulsory if necessary) for the 'normals' on the outside.

Every therapy aims to alter human performance in one way or another. Typically, it is the client's emotional state that is targeted for change, whether directly or by first attending to behaviour, thinking, or memories. However, we do live in a weird world. For example, advertisements by cannibalistic killers for someone to eat so that their respective sexual cravings are satisfied have been answered and followed through (Morrall 2006b). Hence, it might not be too ridiculous to suppose a therapist advertising the augmentation rather than alleviation of despair will find a few customers. But by and large, emotional change through therapy is intended to be in the direction of happiness not misery.

The therapeutic distance travelled towards happiness may be as far as nirvana. Or the trek may only reach 'contentment', 'well-being', or go merely from wretched despair to manageable misery. But, unless the traveller is fortunate to find a Shangri-La, manageable misery is the reality for most people in global society (even if this is presented positively). Moreover, the reality is that the 'therapy culture' is facilitating a futile form of hedonism (Furedi 2003). Being happy is becoming obligatory while global society and the physical planet are in meltdown (Schumaker 2006).

Nirvana

The nuns

Let us now unfrock the nuns (or to put it more respectfully, inspect sceptically research that has been conducted about nuns in relation to happiness). Although nuns are (usually) Catholic Christians, and stereotypically should therefore be riddled with guilt and anguish, some seem to have reached the Buddhist psychological state of ultimate consciousness, harmony, peace, stability, delight, and contentment: Nirvana. Or, if not Nirvana, then a good deal happier than the average commuter struggling through the rush hour to get to work, a parent juggling a career with child-rearing and house-keeping, or a husband/wife negotiating a marriage.

Assessing happiness focuses on subjective reflections rather than scientific measurement. That is, there little or no objectivity in gauging who is happy and who is unhappy. Mostly, what people say about their own emotional condition is what counts as the primary indicator of happiness (or contentment, well-being, and satisfaction). 'Hard' data such as mortality and morbidity rates, living conditions, and material advantage/disadvantage, employment/unemployment, are used, but only in conjunction with personal accounts of emotions. Sophisticated technological procedures, such as placing electrodes into the cerebral cortex and then scanning the brain, is providing interesting information about happiness. But this type of science is only of use if the researcher also knows how the participant is feeling during the procedure (by asking him/her).

Talking to nuns would appear to have been particularly fruitful for those researching into happiness, and is frequently quoted within the happiness literature and used to substantiate the precepts of positive psychology (Seligman 2003). The lifestyles of nuns are based on strict and shared routines. Nuns (at least those from Milwaukee) eat the same food at regular times, conduct the same activities week-by-week, and do not cause researchers major headaches by introducing extraneous variables into their studies by having, for example, exotic holidays, nights out on the town, or flings with the local Don Juan. Leisure excursions, sexual relationships, getting pregnant, marriage, alcohol, and smoking, are either restricted or prohibited. Moreover, nuns tend to have the same access to medical care. However, health and life-span varies considerably within nunneries.

The nun study most often referred to is the longitudinal study over decades of 180 nunnery inmates of the School Sisters of Notre Dame, Milwaukee, Wisconsin, USA. The research involved the nuns writing autobiographical data from early in their twenties into old age (Danner et al. 2001). Most (nearly 60 per cent) had exceeded their expected life-span. But crucially, those who had consistently described positive emotions lived the healthiest and longest. Seemingly, old nuns are happy nuns and happy nuns get old. The researchers suggest that there may be an association between viewing life positively and living a long time because happy people deal with the stresses of life differently to those who are miserable. Positive people do not excite the release of stress-related bio-chemicals (especially cortisol) which are damaging in the long term, particularly to the immune and cardio-vascular system.

However, if the nun researchers *and* John Stuart Mill are right, then the elderly strata of society will always be populated by happy fools.

The bums

After nuns come 'bums' in the study and management of happiness. Extrapolations about the relativity and paradox of happiness have been extrapolated from the results of experiments which entailed probing research participants' rectums (*The Economist*, Editorial, 2006). What Daniel Kahneman, a psychologist and Nobel Prize winner for economics, and his colleagues did was to conduct colonoscopies lasting from just minutes to around an hour (Redelmeier and Kahneman 1996; Redelmeier et al. 2003). Surprisingly, when asked about their experiences, the participants who had been probed for the shorter times reported a higher degree of displeasure than those who had been probed for the longest periods. What appeared to be most significant criteria for the participants in judging their lack of enjoyment about the procedure were the 'worst moments' and 'last moments' rather than duration. A less painful end made the participants happier even if the end was a long time coming.

Kahneman and his co-researchers argue that these rectal experiments show how memory is important for how people view pleasure and displeasure, but that memory is fallible. Extrapolating further, Kahneman suggests that reality is not the important factor in happiness but memories of events that become construed as having been happy. People construct narratives about their lives (for example, regarding their relationships) on the basis of momentous but perhaps momentary happenings. The peaks and finales are remembered above and beyond the totality of the experience. So, a love affair may be recalled as tremendously successful or a horrendous failure because what is retained is the memory of the periods of intense affection or intense aggravation.

The beggars

Since this rectal research, the motion that happiness is relative and paradoxical has been passed repeatedly. Moreover, adding weight to the extrapolations from the nun and bum research is the conclusion drawn from a study of people at the very bottom of the social hierarchy in Calcutta.

Despite an ostensibly squalid and impoverished existence, the homeless, those living in appalling slums, and prostitutes working and living in downmarket brothels, were judged by researcher Robert Diener (2001) to be making the best of a very bad situation. The 83 people he interviewed reported higher levels of well-being than he had expected and one group (the slum dwellers) were nearly as satisfied with their lot in life as the control group of middle-class Calcutta students. Diener conjectured that what made the difference were social relationships. That is, high interpersonal contact and commitment raise the level of satisfaction about an individual's life. Moreover, it helps that the expectation of satisfaction is lower to start with.

Contributing to conclusions from the nun, bum, and beggar studies are the arguments and suggestions of a plethora of social commentators. Incredibly, economists and other social scientists, along with politicians, have found an issue on which they all agree: being rich isn't as good as it seems, and being poor isn't so bad after all.

Conspicuous consumption

Robert Frank (2000), Professor of Management and Professor of Economics at Cornell University, USA, argues that the USA (and by inference the whole of global society) has 'luxury fever'. That is, more and more money is being spent on products that aren't necessary for a happy life. Fast cars, exotic holidays, fashionable clothes, and ever more technological gadgets are bought in the belief that they will provide happiness. They do so briefly, but then their novelty wears off and further luxuries have to be obtained in order to, like an addiction to a drug, get the 'high' again albeit transiently.

Clinical psychologist Oliver James (2007) uses the catchy expression 'affluenza' to describe much the same social process as Frank's 'luxury fever'. However, James argues that the desire to accumulate luxuries has spread like a virus throughout global society. Moreover, turning luxuries into necessities and constant envy about the possessions of others, for James, rather than making people happy, has increased the incidence of mental disorder.

Karl Marx ([1867] 1971), sociologist and economist, well over a hundred years earlier than Frank's and Oliver's analyses, had identified what he termed 'commodity fetishism' which fuels 'conspicuous consumption'. Capitalism at a later stage in its development, he predicted accurately, would require people (consumers) to buy excessively and unnecessarily in order to continue to survive as an economic system. It also has to spread this habit universally, as it is doing with global society becoming a worldwide capitalist market. What Marx wanted, of course, was for capitalism to collapse either through its internal contradictions or revolution. What Frank wants is for people to work fewer hours and enjoy more hobbies. What Oliver wants is for people to stop being so greedy and relax.

Paradox of affluence

Social epidemiologist Richard Wilkinson et al. (2005) argue that throughout the world inequality correlates with life expectancy. However, in societies where inequality is minimal and the society overall is poor (such as Cuba under Fidel Castro), then people are both healthier and happier. In grossly unequal societies (such as the USA under all regimes), the lack of control over work and personal circumstances of those at the bottom of the social hierarchy and knowledge of being at the bottom produce unhealthy habits and low self-esteem which can lead to mental and physical illness, and early death. For Wilkinson and his colleagues, social respect is the key factor. If people receive little or no admiration for the work they do or the money they (don't) have, then they are on the road to destruction. More-over, not only are those in a lower socio-economic position exposed to higher levels of violence and thereby risk an early death, but murder rates correlate with inequality. That is, posits Wilkinson, unfair societies have more murders than poorer ones where the latter have high degrees of social trust. That is, a culture of fairness generates less killing. This phenomenon is true for countries and for sub-sections of a country that have a strong conviction that fairness exists such as particular States in the USA. Redu-cing social exclusion and increased social capital is their answer (that is, increasing interpersonal contact and involvement in civil life).

Underneath much of the commentary and research into the effects of wealth and poverty on happiness is what political writer Gregg Easterbrook (2004) describes as 'The Progress Paradox'. What Easterbrook notes is that in the West wages rose substantially during the twentieth century and people no longer have to be rich to own a house, car, and take holidays abroad regularly. But people are far less happy than would be expected given their relative wealth, and they are frightened.

This is confirmed through sociological research by Glenn Firebaugh and Laura Tach (American Sociological Association 2008). They conclude that after basic needs are satisfied, the degree to which the relative happiness of the wealthy improves depends on comparisons made with the income and possessions of their peers. This comparison with peers means that people place themselves on a 'hedonic treadmill' whereby there is an urge to earn and own more and more.

Easterbrook notes that there is a common cognitive-emotional distortion of 'catastrophizing' among populations of societies in which abundance is prevalent. That is, rather than enjoying and gaining confidence from improvements in employment, health, intelligence, and material ownership, people fear that the worst will happen such as economic collapse or environmental disaster, and also suffer anxiety because of the choices they have. Easterbook wants those who are living in abundance (and wealth is, he argues, spreading globally) to stop whinging about their predicament, accept that their lives are very much better than they would have been a hundred years ago, and be happy!

But merely telling people to be happy may not be enough. Therapy may be needed. Luckily, the ingrates and insane have a rescuer at hand who believes he has the mind technology to settle the paradox of progress, Lord Richard Layard.

Happy economist

Lord Richard Layard is a leading exponent of what he describes as another new science to join the new science of positive psychology: 'happiness economics'. That is, affluent countries have not got much happier as they have grown richer, and, what's more, they are suffering from an increase in mental disorder. Layard agrees that happiness improves only marginally as wealth increase:

> There is a paradox at the heart of our lives. Most people want more income and strive for it. Yet as Western societies have got richer, their people have become no happier ... [W]e have more food, more clothes, more cars, bigger houses, more central heating, more foreign holidays, a shorter working week, nicer work and, above all, better health. Yet we are not happier.
>
> (Layard 2006b: 3)

Layard aims not only to get people off the self-harming hedonic treadmill (what he calls the 'status race'), stop fretfulness, and cure mental disorder into the bargain (2006a).

Layard utilizes research and theories not only from economics, but philosophy, sociology, neuroscience, and psychology (and also refers to the nuns, but not bums or beggars). When being a philosopher, Layard suggests a return to the ideals of the Enlightenment, whereby personal and social happiness are considered the pinnacles of human achievement.

When being a sociologist, he accepts governments must maintain security of work and personal security, and engender trust between people and people and their rulers through the formulation and implementation of specific policies. When being an economist, he is in favour of re-introducing bartering. When being a neuroscientist, he places great faith in evidence from brain scanning which, he argues, demonstrates the direct connection between cerebral activity (in the frontal lobes and amygdala) and feelings. Seemingly, according to the scanners, we can't be happy and unhappy at the same time. When being a psychologist, he wants people to change the way they think and behave, and therefore feel. If people can't get happy by themselves, then positive psychology and cognitive-behavioural therapy should be provided *en masse*.

Happiness and misery can, for Layard, be objectively measured.

Helpfully, Layard offers a definition of what is being measured: 'So by happiness I mean feeling good – enjoying life and wanting the feelings to be maintained. By unhappiness I mean feeling bad and wishing things were different' (Layard 2006b: 12).

Given Layard's prestige as an economist and government adviser, his excursions into philosophy, sociology, neuroscience, and psychology (let alone being a Lord), such a characterization of happiness seems unexpectedly (common) sensible. Layard may wish to formulate a new science about happiness, but he has not yet moved beyond its subjective conceptualization. More worryingly, recommending the availability of therapy on a wide scale (especially the cognitive-behavioural type), is also to foment insidious and politicized personal re-indoctrination.

The goal of nirvana may be laudable but the means to achieve it individualizes the problem: people, not society, are to be 'adjusted'. As Darian Leader (2007) points out, therapies similar to cognitive-behavioural therapy were last used on a mass scale during the 1960s–70s Cultural Revolution in China to alter the views of those whom the Communist politicians and their Red Guard acolytes decided were 'misguided'.

Shangri-La

A programme of cognitive-behavioural therapy aimed at indoctrinating the unhappy masses may not be needed. People are presented continually with self-help guides in the media showing ways to become jolly. Many, of course, have been informed by the research into nuns, bums, and beggars.

For example, Bob Holmes et al. (2003) have produced a ten-point plan to happiness:

1   Earn enough more money (but not excessively so).
2   Desire less.
3   Don't worry if you aren't a genius (as Mill realized, stupid people are more likely to be happy).
4   Make the most of your genetic predisposition towards happiness (pessimists can learn to override their biology and become, if not optimists, then at least less gloomy).
5   Make friends.
6   Stop comparing your physical appearance with others (even if you aren't an 'oil painting' you can convince yourself that you are).
7   Get married (better for men than women, but better than being single for both).

8 Find God (any belief system is good, but preferably ones that aren't into suffering).
9 Be nice to others (it will encourage them to be nice to you).
10 Realize that growing old may not be as bad as you think (elderly people are apparently less despondent about impending death than younger people perceive them to be and more satisfied with their lives than the young).

Alternatively, rather than await re-education, unhappy people could re-locate to Shangri-La. Shangri-La is professed to be a Tibetan community cut off from the rest of the world, a utopian paradise, containing all human knowledge, wisdom, culture, treasures, and can bring contentment to the most discontented of souls. Unfortunately, Shangri-La is fictional. It is a figment of novelist James Hilton's imagination (for his 1933 book *Lost Horizons*).

Iceland, Australia or Vanuatu

So, where on earth could one go to find happiness? Well, there is a country that repeatedly appears at the top of the happiness listings of places to reside. What does that country have that others don't? The topography of this country is mostly unpopulated and infertile plateaus, ice-fields, glaciers, geysers, volcanoes, and hot springs. It has a population of only 3,000,000, has no armed forces, and its economy relies on fishing, aluminium smelting, tourism, and international financing. The climate is mild considering its geographical position, but windy and damp. However, it is nuclear-free, and has one of the highest standards of living in the world when factors of literacy, longevity, income, welfare, wealth distribution, employment rate, and social cohesiveness are taken into account (Central Intelligence Agency 2008a). That country is Iceland.

If Iceland does not suit, then Australia is frequently near the top of 'happy countries' surveys, although there is dispute about whether or not Australians are happy, satisfied, or just well developed as humans (Leigh and Wolfers 2006). If not Iceland or Australia, then a South Pacific island nation that lies between Australia and Hawaii has been also found to be a place of great happiness.

The Happy Planet Index is calculated by examining the relationship between subjective 'life-satisfaction', objective 'life expectancy' and 'environmental impact' (The Happy Planet Index 2006). The first two criteria of the Happy Planet Index are often included in assessments of happiness, but not the third. The impact on the planet's 'happiness' (that is, its ecological healthiness) is contrasted with the means people use to obtain

their person happiness. That is, if a country uses unregulated industrialization and deforestation to raise its people's standard of living (and by
implication their happiness), thereby increasing global pollution and
warming, it gets a low score from the compilers of the Happy Planet Index.
Those countries that have minimal negative impact on the environment and
also furnish happiness include: Iceland, Malta, Austria, Tunisia, Yemen,
Morocco, Palestine, Iran, and São Tome.

Vanuatu (formerly the New Hebrides) tops the list. Its population are
happy *and* environmentally friendly. Comprised of 80 tropical and moun-
tainous islands, only 65 of them are inhabited, and some have active
volcanoes. The population of Vanuatu is approximately 212,000, and its
economy is small-scale agriculture, fishing, offshore financial services, and
tourism. Many of the islands that form Vanuatu are desert-island paradises,
but not utopian and isolated Shangri-Las containing all human knowledge.
Its economy, along with small-scale agriculture and fishing, is made up
partly by the 'knowledge services' of the offshore financial haven variety,
and receives over 60,000 tourists yearly (Central Intelligence Agency
2008b). Consequently, Vanuatu (as with Iceland and Australia) is structurally embedded within global capitalism rather than posing as a substitute
social system.

The Bhutanese

Bhutan also scores very well in the Happy Index in the Happy Planet Index,
which is not surprising given that it has led the way in terms of furnishing a
culture of happiness. Bhutan assesses success through its 'Gross National
Happiness' index instead of the economically driven measurements of
'Gross National Product' and 'Gross Domestic Product'.

Bhutan fits the idea of Shangri-La in many respects. It is a small beautiful
kingdom in the Himalayas between India and China. It only allowed for-
eigners into the country from the 1970s, and continues to restrict the entry
of tourists. Tourism, heavily surcharged, is now providing an effective
source of income. A hereditary monarchy has ruled the country since early
in the twentieth century. The Bhutanese are mainly Buddhists. The population is approximately 672,000. Life expectancy is 63 years for men and
64 years for women. Late in the 1990s television and the internet were
allowed, and King Jigme Khesar Namgyel Wangchuck installed parliamentary democracy in 2008. Introduced in the seventeenth century, the
Bhutanese national dress is the 'gho' for men and 'kira' for women. It is
compulsory.

The 'four pillars' of Bhutan's Gross National Happiness are: (1) the promotion of equitable and sustainable socio-economic development; (2) preservation and promotion of cultural values; (3) conservation of the natural environment; and (4) establishment of good governance (Esty 2004).

Worldwide there are organizations and governments promoting Bhutan's model of how a society should operate. The 'Gross International Happiness Project' (2008) lists the following:

- Bhutan Sustainable Development Secretariat (SDS) and Center of Bhutan Studies, Bhutan
- Spirit in Business, USA and the Netherlands
- Social Venture Network Asia, Thailand
- ICONS, Redefining Progress and Implementing New Indicators on Sustainable Development, Brazil
- Inner Asia Center for Sustainable Development, the Netherlands
- The Government of Mongolia
- The Values Center, USA
- Society for Ecology and Culture, UK and Ladakh, India
- Genuine Progress Indicators, GPI Atlantic, Canada
- New Economics Foundations, UK

But the Gross International Happiness Project with its associated idiosyncratic agencies and minor countries on the world economic and political stage merely serves to underline the fact that most of the world does not follow Bhutan's happiness model.

The mix of happy countries from the different surveys is both surprising and incomprehensive. How can, for example, Kyrgyzstan be compared with Malta, Tunisia with Iceland, Vanuatu with Vietnam, or Australia with Bhutan? Furthermore, such listings of happy countries imply that unhappy people should either move to those registered as happy or their own country should install the culture of a happy country. The leader of the British Conservative Party, David Cameron (2006), has recommended that Britain take up some of the ideals associated with Bhutanese happiness, declaring that 'there is more to life than money', and that social commitment and human contact are better indicators of a happiness than the amount of money someone earns.

Britain, along with the USA, does not appear anywhere near the top of happiness charts. However, both the USA and Britain are inundated with applications for residency and the right to work there, which implies these countries are perceived by those wishing to enter as having the potential to improve their lives. But, moving to another country, certainly in the short term, undermines rather than bolsters our happiness, because of the loss of social capital. Social capital is considered to be paramount in raising happiness levels in society (Wilkinson et al. 2005).

Cyberspace and architecture

Could cyberspace offer a mid-route between the fictional Shangri-La and moving to Bhutan? Professor Robert Putman of Public Policy at Harvard University, USA, is a happiness expert who also believes in social capital as a key source of happiness (2004; 2006). He is sceptical about social capital being nurtured electronically (and is very critical of the effects of television on social capital). For him virtual communities do not replace the quality of real human interaction. He does accept that where electronic communication leads to actual face-to-face contact (for example, through the use of internet dating sites), there's a positive outcome for social capital and thereby happiness.

Instead of moving to a Bhutan-style Shangri-La, changing one's own society to the Bhutan model, or living in the happy regions of cyberspace, it might be easier to relocate houses or redesign the house lived in presently. Philosopher Alain de Botton has studied how architecture affects emotions (de Botton 2006). He sees some buildings as 'angst-ridden'. One fast-food outlet in particular disgusts him: a McDonald's in London. London's Westminster Cathedral, however, seemingly makes him happy, as does his own home.

False comparisons

But as Michael Bond (2003) argues, Bhutan is not a major Western country with a well-developed capitalist economy. Indeed, it is culturally isolated and impoverished. How would it therefore be possible to transfer the lifestyle of the Bhutanese and replace economic measures with those of happiness when capitalist societies are essentially driven by their economies? This is an observation made by Marx ([1867] 1971). The cultures of *all* types of economic systems are driven by the nature of their economies. Furthermore, the global advancement of capitalism means that countries such as Bhutan will be left behind economically and culturally. Bond also points out that there are defining nuances between different capitalist countries in relation to happiness. Rampant individualism is part of the culture of some capitalist countries (such as Britain and the USA), and personal achievement is what makes people happy. In other capitalist counties which are more collectivist such as Japan, China and South Korea, people are more fatalistic towards happiness (not being happy is not seen as a personal failure but more the responsibility of society), and also less likely to gain social respect from personal achievement.

It is unrealistic for global society to alter the forces of capitalism and take up a Bhutanese Shangri-La, no-matter how attractive that might appear in terms of improving happiness. The reality is capitalism is expanding, not retracting. Consumerism, globalization, private ownership, and the cult of the individual are raging worldwide. Bhutan is much more likely to falter in its attempt to forestall these forces than the other way around. In any event, it is highly improbable that the Bhutanese national dress will be adopted elsewhere, unless as a fashion item within an economic system that is happy to commodify anything.

Reality

There is a far starker reality, however, than recognizing that the Bhutanese style of happiness and national dress would be difficult to disseminate. That is, the presence of deprivation, disease, disaster, and danger for so many people in the world. It is not happiness that millions of people desire, it is survival.

Moreover, can the private troubles that bring individuals to therapy equate to the troubles of global society? Should so many resources be spent on the personal misery or on improving happiness when every day children and adults die unnecessarily?

Global problems

The United Nations (2008a) has compiled a list of the social 'issues' in the world from which it formulates an agenda for action both by its own personnel, other non-government agencies, and governments. It includes:

- Africa
- Ageing
- AIDS
- Climate Change
- Disarmament
- Drugs and Crime
- Education
- Elections
- Energy
- Environment
- Food

- Governance
- Health
- Human Rights
- Humanitarian and Disaster Relief Assistance
- Indigenous People
- Intellectual Property
- International Finance
- International Law
- Iraq
- Law of the Sea and Antarctica
- Least Developed Countries
- Outer Space
- Peace and Security
- Persons with Disabilities
- Population
- Question of Palestine
- Refugees
- Sustainable Development
- Terrorism
- Water
- Women

The divide between the wealthy minority and impoverished majority is growing. The ecological and material self-interest of the Western world and the major industrializing countries, along with the equally self-serving and corrupt actions of the economic and political elites in under-developed countries, has created a polarized world population.

Late in 2006, the World Institute for Development Economics Research (WIDER) of the United Nations University reported that 10 per cent of the richest adults in the world owned 85 per cent of global household wealth (WIDER 2006). Davies et al. (2006) recorded that the richest 2 per cent of adults in the world own more than half of all household wealth, and the poorer half own less than 1 per cent.

Global warming and pollution may, without recuperative strategies being employed urgently, tip the earth into a spiral of unrecoverable environmental collapse characterized by droughts, famines, floods, and tsunamis (Gore 2006; Klobert 2006; Lovelock 2006).

Violence is endemic, and the global murder rate per annum is rising toward one million (Morrall 2006a, 2007a). The International Institute for Strategic Studies reports on 70 recently resolved, in abeyance, or ongoing armed conflicts (2008). Armed conflicts through external wars, civil unrest, border disputes, insurgency, and terrorism during 2006–2007 included: Algeria, Burma, China, Colombia, Democratic Republic of the Congo, India/Pakistan, Kosovo, Indonesia, Georgia, Israel, Palestinian Territories, Côte d'Ivoire (Ivory Coast), North Korea, Nepal, Democratic Republic of Timor-Leste (East Timor), Nigeria, Peru, Philippines, Russia, Chechnya, Somalia, Ethiopia, Iraq, United States, Britain, Sri Lanka, Uganda, Thailand, Uzbekistan, Yemen, Eritrea, Serbia, Turkey, Afghanistan, Lebanon, Morocco/Western Sahara, Spain, Liberia, Cyprus, Haiti, and Sudan. The budget for peacekeeping operations by the United Nations in the year 2006–2007 was US$5.28 billion to deal with 16 conflicts, with US$41.54 billion having been spent between 1944–2006, and a further US$1.90 still owed (United Nations 2008b).

Life expectancy

Japanese, Icelanders, Israelis, Norwegians, Swedes, Britons, Italians, Germans, French, Canadians, Australians, and Singaporeans are living to around 80 years of age (although citizens of the USA, the wealthiest and most powerful country on earth, has a lower life expectancy of 77.5 years). Millions of people in Sub-Saharan countries have lower life expectancies than the working classes of England in the 1840s. Rwandans will probably only live for the first few years of their fourth decade, Malawis and Angolans will likely just get to 40, Zambians will be extremely lucky if they reach 40 years, and being a native of Swaziland means that you will probably die at just over 30 years (United Nations 2006).

Some sub-regions and substrata of countries, which overall have respectable life-span profiles, contain populations which on average die at significantly younger ages (for example, shanty-towns of Brazil; blacks in the southern states of the USA; peasants in Indo-China; the Aborigenes of Australia; industrial workers in the 'Special Economic Zones' of the People's Republic of China).

Early death in the under-developed world is the result of specific and inter-related factors: (1) disease (for example, as a consequence of HIV/AIDS, malaria, and smoking); (2) poverty (associated with: environmental catastrophe; unfair Western-orientated trading arrangements; home-grown political corruption and financial incompetence, and warfare); and (3) accidents (related to unregulated working conditions, and dangerous transport infrastructure).

Within developed countries wide disparities in longevity mean that the executive, management, and white-collar classes in such countries as Britain and the USA live longer than those with menial jobs and those in the underclass. The reasons for the latter groups dying younger – perhaps up to ten years – can be categorized in the same way as in the under-developed world: (1) disease (principally: cancers; cerebro-vascular trauma; cardio-vascular disorder); (2) poverty (associated with unemployment, long-term physical or mental illness, and homelessness); and (3) accidents (for example, mishaps at work, on the roads, and in the home).

Infant/child mortality

A similar pattern to that of longevity is apparent in the statistics for infant and under-5 deaths. Infant mortality per 1,000 births in a year in Somalia is 126 and under-5 mortality 211, Afghanistan 149 and 252, Niger 154 and 264, and Occupied Palestinian Territory 21 and 24 (United Nations 2006). In Australia, Italy, Israel, and the United Kingdom it is 5 and 6 respectively, Germany 4 and 6, France and Norway 4 and 5, Iceland, Sweden, and Singapore and Japan 3 and 4. The USA rates are 7 and 8 (United Nations 2006).

Hundreds of millions of children either do not attend school or receive inadequate schooling. One in four adults in the developing world is illiterate. Nearly a billion people are undernourished. Nearly a billion people do not have access to proper health care. Over a billion do not have access to safe drinking water (World Revolution 2008).

Summary

To be happy when the world is in such a mess, or worse, to try to make those not directly involved in the mess happier, is duplicitous. Moreover, advising those who are not as happy as they would like to be *because* their life is relatively safe, secure, plentiful, to consume happiness while billions of others are hungry, diseased, maimed, exploited, and destroyed, is moral madness.

Happiness has actually been considered to be madness. Richard Bentall (1992) proposes (ironically) that happiness should be classified as a mental disorder. For him, the obsessive searching for happiness is a disorder of emotion, which he labelled 'major affective disorder: pleasant type'. Bentall predicts (tongue in cheek) that 'happiness clinics' should be set up and 'anti-happiness medication' prescribed.

I suggest (with no irony and my tongue firmly out of my cheek) that the promotion of happiness is responsible for 'false hope syndrome: unpleasant type'. That is, therapists, together with positive psychologists and the merchants of self-help, are deceiving people into believing that authentic and durable alterations in human happiness are possible by re-training the mind to be optimistic. The happiness industry is successful commercially and ideologically because consumers of happiness misinterpret their failure to be upbeat. The hyped promises detailed in happiness products, and the initial victories over misery, override doubt about the possibility for emotional change. As Janet Polivy explains:

> People appear to behave paradoxically, by persisting in repeated self-change attempts despite previous failures. It is argued, though, that self-change attempts provide some initial rewards even when unsuccessful. Feelings of control and optimism often accompany the early stages of self-modification efforts. In addition, unrealistic expectations concerning the ease, speed, likely degree of change, and presumed benefits of changing may overwhelm the knowledge of one's prior failures. It is thus important to learn to distinguish between potentially feasible and impossible self-change goals in order to avoid overconfidence and false hopes leading to eventual failure and distress.
>
> (Polivy 2001: 80)

Furthermore, much of the happiness industry is underpinned by a 'new science'. But this 'new science' is pseudoscience. Happiness research although 'scientized', has been founded on highly selective groups (nuns, beggars, and Bhutanese), and peculiar penetration of the body. Also, inappropriate cross-cultural comparisons are proffered, and outrageous (over-)generalizations been made about what happiness is, and what can be done about unhappiness. Crucially, this 'science' accepts for the most part that what people say happiness is can be considered as reality. Such subjectivity cannot be generalized. My happiness may not be your happiness (or anyone else's).

Another sceptical consideration is that there has been a shift from enduring misery as an integral and important element of the human condition or a hallowed totem of religiosity, to the 'demiseryization' of society. Demiseryization is a form of psycho-social cleansing whereby the individual and ultimately society have discomfort and despair anaesthetized or eradicated. The removal of misery, however, not only reduces our own humanity but also human empathy. Not to have experienced psychological pain (or indeed physical pain) disallows compassion as we cannot appreciate the pain of others.

But it's not just the research methods of the new 'science' that are flaky. Some of the principal architects of the new science have borrowed their theoretical foundations from the scientifically controversial discipline of evolutionary psychology. For positive psychologist Martin Seligman (2006) and evolutionary psychologist Daniel Nettle (2005), evolution has steered human brain functioning and human performance towards negativity. Humans are never satisfied with what they have got, and all too readily jump on the 'hedonic treadmill'. Our 'catastrophic' brain is preparing for future danger, and therefore enjoying what is present is not an option. The 'trick of nature' is that we crave happiness but work against ourselves in the attempt to be happy. So what can counteract hundreds of thousands of years of self-imposed biologically impregnated misery? Apparently, short-term therapies and such exercises as identifying our strengths, filling in a daily 'gratitude diary', and writing letters to those people to whom we owe a debt of thanks and reading them out to them rather than sending them by post.

But this evolutionary explanation has major contradictions. According to the happiness theorists, many people are happy without being on the hedonic treadmill. Also, the perceptions of the enlightened are not distinguished from those of the unenlightened by these happiness theorists. To paraphrase John Stuart Mill, I'd rather be a miserable thinker than a happy fool. Moreover, it is Mill who points to the immorality of concentrating only on individualized happiness: '[T]hat [moral] standard is not the agent's own personal happiness, but the greatest amount of happiness altogether' (Mill [1861] 2001). Perhaps, in praise of grumpiness, the strategy to improve collective human happiness should be filling in 'ingratitude diaries', writing letters of complaint to all those who can make a difference in the world and demand they listen to them being read out, and undergo anti-false-hope syndrome and/or 'ranting therapy' to raise and express our consciousness and consciences for what Mill calls the 'greatest happiness principle' and thereby defeat the 'great deceit'.

Some people, however, reverse the process of moving from unenlightenment to enlightenment. Heather did just that.

Heather's raised consciousness about her vacuous happiness meant that, after one or two false starts, she had gone to university, gained a first-class degree, and become a teacher. However, her raised consciousness also made her realize that she would have to continue to make enormous efforts for her self-development to be such that she could reach authentic and durable happiness. On that realization, she returned to self-deception about happiness, and reemployed the deceitful strategy of choosing partners she considered capable of 'making her happy'. What she consciously sought were partners who could provide substantial emotional support (and if they brought with them financial collateral, all the better). Self-responsibility together with collective responsibility was simply too much hard work for Heather, and her feelings of insecurity and rejection too potent, for her to seek to be happy (in the enlightened sense) by her own means and to bestow happiness spontaneously and unconditionally on others.

Conclusion

Review

Redemption

Heather

Review

The trouble with therapy is that it is 'asocial'. The therapeutic enterprise pays scant attention to the mess in global society. Moreover, it is socially atavistic. The therapeutic enterprise today exists in a primitive form, characterized by dysfunctionality, arrogance, selfishness, abusiveness, infectiousness, insanity, and deceit.

That is, therapeutic enterprise is institutionally splintered, and undergoing therapy is a gamble. Science is increasingly being used to justify the efficacy of therapy. But there is over-confidence in the promotion of 'scientific therapies' as confidence in science itself can be called into question.

Therapy focuses on the 'self' and in doing so individualizes suffering that actually has its roots in society. Therapy ignores social conceptualizations of the self and how the self is changing rapidly in global society (for example, becoming sexualized and saturated). There is inadequate appreciation by therapists of how personal power is affected by social power, and of how the therapeutic enterprise is an agency of social control, particularly through its association with the 'sick role'.

Therapists are responsible for the spreading of a new social disease – 'therapyitis'. More and more therapy means people become less and less able to sort out 'problems with living' for themselves, and governments avoid taking responsibility for those issues which are social in origin. Therapy deals with, but is uneducated about, madness. This lack of knowledge about madness covers both medical and sociological conceptualizations. Such ignorance *is* madness.

Inequality, disease, pollution, and violence are intractable realities for much of the world's population. For economist Paul Collier (2007), the reality for the 'bottom billion' of the twenty-first-century global society is that the conditions are more identifiable with the fourteenth century. Notwithstanding that level of social suffering, the therapeutic enterprise, along with the 'positive' branch of psychology and the trade in self-help commodities, promulgate a delusional version of personal happiness.

But is formal therapy any better than friendship? That old troublemaker Jeffrey Masson (1990) makes the accusation that therapy is a 'corruption of friendship'. The client is offered a relationship that may appear to be a friendship, in that he/she is encouraged to share his/her closest secrets and feelings, but this in reality is a false friendship. The relationship is between a (so-called) professional and a client, and the reason they meet is for the respective purposes of 'selling' and 'consuming' a service, not simply because they like each other.

For Masson, what is needed to help people with their psychological distress, are more kindly friends and fewer formal therapists. The re-installation in society of 'kindly friendliness' as a valued human quality with a valuable social function means that the role of therapy in society would become either restricted or obsolete. However, in a commodified and consumerized global market, 'kindly friendliness' would soon be packaged and sold in high street stores and on the internet. Within only a few years, 'kindly friendliness' would have representative agencies with regulatory authority, and the cycle of professionalizing a 'natural' human and social phenomenon would begin again.

The relationship of Heather (this book's resident client) and her barefoot therapist, Len (a kindly friend who also has the basic skills of therapy) contained falsehoods. They had strayed from friendship, to an informal client–therapist relationship, and then to lovers, blurring each into the other whenever the need arose. It would not be unusual for the naked sexual engagement of these friends to spill over into bare therapeutic interchanges, all in one evening.

But the mixing of sexuality, love and friendship, does occur in formal therapy, either as part of the 'issue' the client brings to therapy or within the client–therapist relationship. Prostitution also entangles sex, love, friendship, with (barefoot) therapy. Veronica Monet claims to have had sex with a couple of thousand men during her career as an 'escort', and has written about her experiences (Monet 2005). Monet records that many of her clients enjoyed not only the sex but also the 'friendship' they formed with the prostitutes. According to Monet, the men gained not only physical but psychological release from the conversations they had with the women. Monet was the archetypal 'tart with a heart'.

David Smail argues that, no matter how diluted, love is being exchanged in therapy. Certainly, the precepts of humanistic therapy are closely associated with conditions of love (trust, honesty, unconditional regard, and genuineness). Moreover, although genital contact is virtually universally proscribed within therapy (the exception being Wilhelm Reich's 'Orgone Therapy': Reich 1989), some degree of sexual tension is common to many forms of intensive interpersonal contact.

For Jeffrey Schaler (1995), therapy and prostitution are much the same except that prostitutes are more sincere than therapists. The client is rarely fooled by the degree of care on offer from a prostitute, but clients are frequently unaware that therapists are only pretending to care for their clients. Therefore, not only is therapy immoral because it ignores the mess of global society, but as Schaler agues, it is immoral in its pretence of friendship.

Redemption

But therapy is not beyond redemption. Sociological enlightenment can be incorporated into the therapeutic enterprise to extricate itself from its asocial and atavistic predicament. There is an equivalent task for a trouble-making sceptical therapist to enlighten sociology.

The sociological imagination and sociological theories offer a broader appreciation of human problems than does therapy, and a sceptical dissection of how the therapeutic enterprise operates in society. Humans and their social environment cannot be detached. Human problems, for the sociologist, are either born of society or have a strong connection to society. Private troubles are social issues, and social issues cause private troubles.

The effect of the social-environmental on private troubles is appreciated by Oliver James (2008). Although not a 'therapist' in the sense I have been using that term here (he is a clinical psychologist, as well as author, media broadcaster, and political adviser), James is more sociologically enlightened than most in the field of psychological distress (helped no doubt by studying social anthropology at university). He regards 'selfish capitalism' as damaging to human well-being, particularly the variety extolled by English-speaking nations which promotes unfettered and toxic materialism, and creates huge divisions between the rich and the poor. It is this variety that is presently contaminating much of the rest of the world. James does not recommend fervent insurrection to destroy the social, political, and economic structures and processes of selfish capitalism. Instead, he believes that the solution is 'simple': 'Instead of continuing with Selfish Capitalism, our politicians must start the work of persuading us to adopt the unselfish variety' (James 2008: 230). Sooner or later, James postulates, this solution will become the programme of a political party or political leader.

I agree with James's analysis of 'selfish capitalism' but not his optimism about the inevitability of, nor proclivity for, 'unselfish capitalism'. Indeed, as structural sociology demonstrates, capitalism (whether selfish or unselfish) is by its very nature exploitative. There have to be financial winners and losers within any capitalist system, and capitalism is always driven by consumerism and commodification.

Therapists have a social responsibility not just to be *analytical* (although that would be a good starting point) but to be *actively* troublesome. Together with sociologists, therapists should be working *passionately* for the production and implementation of *radical* policies and allegiances designed to clean up the mess in global society. This could lead to sociology and therapy (along with professional and academic disciplines such as psychology, science, and medicine) uniting and collaborating with other humanitarian agencies to tackle the reality of misery in global society by fermenting as much trouble (both analysis *and* action) as possible. Without this sociologically enlightened analytical and activist edge to therapy, it becomes part of the problem, not the solution to the troubles of the world. Concentrating on the microcosm of human suffering means that macroscopic suffering is not understood and not dealt with. The problems of poverty, plague, pestilence, and pitilessness, become secondary to problems with boyfriends, boredom, and blame. Hiccoughs in everyday human existence are being indulged while the death-rattle of social life is being ignored.

However, some therapists do propose macrocosmic solutions to the problems of global society (for example, Pilgrim 1997; Proctor et al. 2006; Totton 2006). These few radicals are raising their sights from the circumscribed navel-gazing of therapy, looking above the parapet of self-indulgence, and arguing for social responsibility *and* social change to be part of the therapeutic enterprise.

Andrew Samuels (2006) refers to a number of therapy organizations that have social agendas. For example, 'Psychotherapists and Counsellors for Social Responsibility' assists therapists to intervene in political matters. The 'St James's Alliance' aims to politicize psychological, ethical and spiritual concerns in society. Apart from therapists, it consists of representatives from politics, economics, ethics, religion, non-governmental organizations, activist and pressure groups, and the media:

> Psychotherapists, along with economists, social scientists, religious people, environmentalists and others, can contribute to a general transformation of politics. Today's politicians leave many with a sense of deep despair and disgust. They seem to lack integrity, imagination and new ideas. Across the globe and in response to the challenge, a search is on to remodel politics. Psychotherapy's contribution to this search depends on opening a two-way street between inner realities and the world of politics. We need to balance attempts to understand the secret politics of the inner world of emotional, personal and family experiences with the secret psychology of pressing outer world matters such as leadership, the economy, environmentalism, nationalism and war.
>
> (Samuels 2006: 4)

I do not have the solution to the mess of the world. Nor do I believe that a conglomeration of therapists, sociologists, psychologists, medical practitioners, scientists, and humanitarians, would have either. Any convention held by such an alliance may turn out more like a hippie festival than a vanguard of proto-revolutionaries, and 'beating the drum for social change' could become less of a metaphor and more of literal exercise to facilitate 'togetherness'. However, it would be a start. Millions work in the health, mind, social, and caring industries, science, and academia. Collectively, they have the potential to be a powerful social movement (with or without drums).

My input to such a convention would be to recommend 'simple' solutions:

1   'Global Government for Global Society' (with representation from: national and cross-national ethnic, religious/spiritual, humanist,

humanitarian, environmental, media, sporting, leisure/entertainment, and animal rights groups; and international scientific/academic and occupational disciplines).

2 'Health not Wealth' (the driving ideology for humanity should be its physical, emotional, spiritual, cultural, and environmental, well-being; while respecting cultural diversity, moral universals are defined and propagated; 'wealth' becomes a consequence of, not catalyst for, civilized human life).

3 'From Social Atavism to Social Actualization' (the present time-warp of social life to be given a momentous jolt, first, by accepting that it still is 'uncivilized', and, second, by recognizing that achieving personal or social satisfaction is not trouble-free – humans have to strive to thrive).

My suggestions for modifying if not eradicating dysfunctionality, arrogance, selfishness, abusiveness, infectiousness, insanity, and deceit, from therapy are:

1 *Dysfunction*: the mandatory setting-up of national therapy agencies similar to the British General Medical Council; working towards the creation of a global therapy agency, with regional/local sub-agencies.

2 *Selfishness*: a shift away from 'the self' as the only locus of attention during therapy towards a dialogue with the client's 'social self' (that is a self that includes due deference to personal *and* social factors, and interventions are thereby sociologically informed).

3 *Arrogance*: the limitations of scientific evidence should be expressed in therapy literature; non-empirical, but otherwise rational epistemologies can be accommodated within the therapeutic enterprise.

4 *Infectiousness*: lessons must be learned from both the success and downside of professionalized medicine; professionalization should be abandoned as an irrelevant occupational strategy in favour of 'skilled worker' status; 'skilled therapists' should be identified as having a restricted but well-developed range of attributes that have specified applications (fashionable, asocial, and 'crazy' therapies should be excluded); barefoot therapy, as with informal care for physical health, must remain the option of first choice for resolving personal troubles.

5 *Insanity*: all therapy training curricula to include a thorough explication of medical and sociological knowledge about psychological distress/madness.

6 *Deceit*: all therapy training curricula to include sociological knowledge; therapy must be de-coupled from the commercialization of human happiness; the legitimization of rigorous and forthright debates about society to be held at every opportunity (for example, in all therapy

conferences); 'impossibilism' to be tackled (that is, the notion that nothing can be done about global suffering should be challenged); vigorous and committed alignments made between agencies of therapy and ethical causes with the express aim of alleviating global misery; therapy and sociology to align strategically for the benefit of both, and engage in political analysis *and* action.

Heather

Heather's story has unquestionably helped me to formulate this troublesome and sceptical sociological review of therapy. Exploring her story in this book has grounded my thinking and forced me to consider how real people with real troubles might be helped or hindered by therapy.

This is an unusual technique for sociologists. Sociologists are prone to inhabit an abstract macrocosmic explanatory zone that bears little to the experience of most people, just as therapists are far too near the concrete microcosmic zone of everyday human issues. The former cannot see the wood for the trees whereas the latter cannot see the trees for the wood. There is, therefore, reciprocal benefit for therapy and sociology in joining forces. A specific example from my own research has been the usefulness of psychoanalytic concepts when digging into the roots of the fascination with murder (Morrall 2006a).

There is no conclusion to Heather's story, happy or otherwise. Neither Len nor I know much about what happened to Heather. True to her guise as Dr Jekyll and Mr Hyde, a few hours after Len had received by text this message from Heather, 'I wish with all my heart that you could be here to come home to, to laugh and to love with. I will always love you', he received another and final message, 'It's all over'.

In a state of emotional numbness, Len responded in a feeble whisper to himself with Leonard Cohen's poignant lyric 'Hey, that's no way to say goodbye'.[1] Once the autonomic protective mind-anaesthesia had worn off, he was to wallow interminably in the sentiments of that song.

Up until that point Len believed Heather had been faithful to him, give or take a night or two. Len, with anger and injured pride perhaps still clouding his opinion, believes that his therapeutic usefulness to Heather had run out, as had his role as her father-figure and partner, and that she had for some time being planning her exit from their relationship. He surmised that her sudden and emphatic elimination of him from her life was linked directly to his demand that *his* needs, wants, dreams, and hopes, had to be taken into consideration, and because he had been open about *his* insecurities and fears of rejection. As a consequence of these demands and openness, Heather had, according to Len, wrongly deduced that his commitment to and love for her were shaky. But he had never held a woman that close.

What Len did discover from a third party was that not long after sending the text tersely terminating their relationship, she had moved on to, and moved in with, the man who became her (next) husband. The globalized commodification of everything had allowed another consumer of relationships to dispose of an unwanted lover either to be recycled in the market of human love or buried in the landfill site of broken hearts. Before discarding this one, however, Heather had been astute enough to select and trial the prospective human goods, and ensure it came with a better guarantee.

After five years of being Heather's friend, barefoot therapist, and lover, followed by a long period of reflection, Len thinks he has come to understand some but not all of Heather's persona. He is fully aware that others could provide alternative accounts. Moreover, it would be fascinating to know Heather's version of *her* story.

But, given an assumed bias to and limits of Len's version, and missing corroborating evidence, what is known about this 'client' is massively more than is usually disclosed during therapy. Knowledge gained by a formal therapist about any client cannot compete with the intensity and longevity of Len and Heather's relationship. Len spent thousands of hours talking with Heather about her life, past, needs, wants, dreams, and hopes, listening, advising, challenging, and supporting her, and working to make her smile.

Whether a perfunctory 'quickie', indulgently introspective, or idealistically empathic therapy, and no matter how superior the therapeutic skills and qualities of the therapist, 'certified helping' can only be a shabby replica of help given by a committed and capable barefoot therapist. A course of 50-minute sessions, whether numbering six or sixty, cannot replicate the information and understanding of a friend, relative, or lover who has known the 'client' for years if not a lifetime, particularly if he/she has at least rudimentary communicative abilities.

This is especially so as therapy has only reached its occupational adolescence compared to, for example, medicine's relative maturity. The equivalent in health care to the dedicated and insightful significant other helping to resolve private troubles, is folk, traditional, and complementary/ alternative healers. But the barefoot doctor is not a huge threat to the status of the scientific doctor, unlike the barefoot therapist to the formal therapist. Medicine has the social power of a fully-fledged profession, whereas therapy is struggling to find a unified discourse and representative agency, as well as dominance and autonomy over private troubles.

Crucially, Len, as well as being a participant in parts of Heather's life, is a journalist and therefore relatively socially aware. He can place at least some of her performance within its social context. Len, as not only a barefoot therapist but a barefoot sociologist, is cognizant of the effect of structural conditions, how personal meanings are garnered from social interactions, and how the constructions of postmodern society affect the family, the role of women, the world of education and work, and lifestyles generally.

It is the premise of this book that therapists are not so well informed, and that the weaknesses of the therapeutic enterprise, like those of Heather, stop it from rising to play a greater part in global society.

What Len did not know about Heather was exactly what had happened in her childhood, what had occurred between her and her father, and exactly what the mix of nature and nurture, had caused the troubled facets of her persona (the dysfunction, arrogance, abusiveness, selfishness, infectiousness, delusion, and insanity). But what he did grasp in due course was that her persona was a simulation of global society, both 'messed up' and 'muddling through' the mess. Furthermore, Heather's Mr Hyde traits were outweighed by her Dr Jekyll qualities. Len believed that although it would take years she would eventually cross her lines of self-defence. She then could rise to play a greater part in resolving her feeling of insecurity and rejection, and become less troubled and troublesome.

Len also came to question *his* self and *his* performance through the telling of Heather's story. Why had Len persevered with Heather? What was he gaining from an association which listed so markedly to one side that it threatened to drown him in a sea of emotional despair and destructiveness? Was he unwittingly and inescapably caught in the grip of Heather's emotional undertow, or could he have at any time swum to the safe sands of emotional stability by simply leaving her? Why had he allowed himself to give so much without receiving much in return? Was there a psychological pay-off for Len from placing himself willing in the role of the injured party? Why did he allow himself to be persuaded by Heather to re-enter their relationship after it had on so many occasions collapsed, and so energetically pursue its reformation when eventually it was terminated permanently by Heather? After receiving little from their connection, how is it that he was so devastated when it had gone forever? In his words, 'his heart had been murdered'. But some victims of 'murder' share complicity for their demise with their killers (Morrall 2006a).

From bitter searching of his bitter heart, Len knew he was not completely innocent. Len's lament was that Heather had not understood that he had adored her, had always been there for her, and had offered her those aspects of himself that he thought were of use in the struggle she had with her self.

On first meeting, Heather and Len's conversations centred on her desire to 'grow' and be more 'fulfilled'. Having made such a journey in life himself, Len had sincerely and conscientiously encouraged Heather to achieve whatever she thought might be a more satisfying way to live her life. Len regarded the bicycling journey they took together up a very long and extremely steep hill on an exceptionally hot and humid day as a metaphor for 'thriving through striving'. Moreover, he had thought it an indication of a growing friendship that might become mutually fulfilling. They had succeeded in cycling to the pinnacle of the hill through their individual physical tenacity *and* the emotional sustenance from being a couple.

But Len also has his Hyde side, and perhaps much of his negative alto-ego was a mirror to Heather's Hyde. He could be a devil and as much an angel. They were, Heather was to remark, like 'two little Hitlers'[2] fighting for dominance, each blaming the other for their interpersonal atrocities.

There are many avenues for therapists attempting to answer Len's questions to meander down, and help Len 'come to terms with' his devastation. Humanists might want to 'be with' Len in the present, psychoanalytic/psychodynamic therapists may wish to visit similar incidents in his past, and cognitive-behaviourists may try to alter his 'faulty' thinking. Therapists enlightened by sociology may combine their chosen approach with illuminations, for example, about the 'construction' and 'sickness' of love, the fluidity of emotions and the self in society, and the structural pressures and freedoms that encourage or discourage human relationships (Giddens 2006; Turner 2007; Tallis 2005).

The trouble with Len (and Leonard Cohen) is that he could find no cure for love, and his only therapy was for her to walk by him again[3].

Notes

Introduction

1   I use 'therapy' as a generic term for counselling and psychotherapy unless the issue under discussion demands a distinction to be made. I am also consistently referring to 'talking' therapies. Excluded, therefore are approaches that involve primarily such non-talk techniques as art, music, or play.

2   This is an adaptation of an expression offered to me by a trained therapist (who also happens to be an ex-wife) for the model learned during these summer schools.

3   Real-estate agent or realtor.

4   The retelling of an in-joke between Heather and her friend and barefoot therapist Len cannot do it justice: Heather's spontaneous invention of 'arm-rustling' (the vigorous jerking of upper-limb adipose tissue in the attempt to make a noise) when challenged to 'arm-wrestling' by Len, for reasons that relate to their perpetual mutual competitiveness, was at the time nothing short of inspirational comedic improvisation.

1 Enlightenment

1 I have borrowed and extended Erving Goffman's concept of 'performance', which is connected to his view that humans live their life as if in a 'drama' Goffman 1959), as a shorthand description for the range of 'things' that make humans human. 'Performance' as it is used here encompasses (a) human behaviours (what humans do physically, for example, run for a bus; cry; laugh; yell; write; travel; punch; have sex); (b) human thinking (the cognitive processes that involve, for example, imagination; concentration; intelligence; and reflection); and (c) human emotions (the feeling that are precursors to or outcomes of thinking and behaviour such as rage, love, indifference, happiness, and misery.

2 No 'body of knowledge' in the natural or social sciences can profess epistemological fusion; the division of knowledge into 'natural' and 'social' (or 'science' and art) is arbitrary; moreover, so far searches for a coalescing 'theory of everything' have not only proven fruitless but counter-productive.

3 For example, most electronic forms of newspapers carry large numbers of 'pop-up' advertisements to compensate for the loss of revenue caused by falling 'hard-copy' sales.

4 Although metals, planets, protons, neutrons, grass, and air do not have a reflective consciousness, the 'intelligent design' of objects is theoretically feasible (perhaps by the mating of neurons with silicon circuits to produce bio-computers).

5 The discrepancy in usage between therapy and sociology is a good example of what Weber is getting at when he points out that 'knowledge' – such as empathy – has unique conditions and histories – such as those associated with therapy versus those coming from sociology – which affect its meaning.

6 My thanks goes to Dee Cooper, therapist, who many years ago drew my attention to the significance of *La Nausée*.

7 My thanks to the Reverend Alan Brown, friend and colleague at the University of Leeds, who repeatedly reminds me that we do indeed 'live in a messy world' to combat my attempts at rational explanations for what appear to be contradictory aspects of human performance.

2 Dysfunctional

1 An example of excellent *and* straightforward text that explores theories and practices is Colin Feltham and Ian Horton's (2005) *The Sage Handbook of Counselling and Psychotherapy*; an example of an excellent and straightforward text that explores theories and practices *and* which, exceptionally, includes a degree of sociology is John McLeod's (2003) *An Introduction to Counselling*.

2 I have avoided using acronyms or abbreviations for most of the organizations

referred to in this chapter so as to avoid confusion (particularly as some organizations have the same acronym).

3   Could there be a case for 'irrational'-emotive therapy? Theorists with such disparate backgrounds as the Freudian-Marxist Erich Fromm (1963) and the phenomenological-existentialist R. D. Laing (1965), have argued that it is the client's social context that is 'irrational' rather than the client him/herself. Consequently, a more realistic therapeutic intervention might be to confront 'rational' connections between thinking, emotions, and behaviour as such rationality can only be illusion.

4   The type of psychodynamic therapy titled 'intensive' can be deceptive as it may mean either lots of sessions during a short period of time (for example, three a week over six weeks), or, as with psychoanalysis, each session is highly contemplative (and the duration of therapy extensive).

5   It might be interesting – and fun – to test out a 'perverse therapy' which encapsulates insensitivity, suspicion, pretension, and duplicity, given that most human relationships contain these negative elements; such a therapeutic relationship, therefore would be more realistic.

6   The British Association for Counselling does not publicize the full list of its member organizations.

3   Arrogant

1   Research by Szasz and Hollender (1956) into doctor–patient relationships indicated that for much of the time medical consultations were founded on the patient being passive and the doctor being active. I suggest that Szasz and Hollender's model has application to the client–therapist role.

2   This is a phrase I have borrowed from Jürgen Habermas (1975) who applied it to the political sphere.

3   Given that American English is employed in this book, then presumably its scope is intended to be wider that just a British audience.

4   On its website (accessed 25 June 2007), the Harvard Center for Cancer Prevention, Harvard School of Public Health uses a summary of evidence about multivitamins relating to cancer collated until 2005.

4   Selfish

1   To remind the reader, I use the term 'performance' to describe the feelings, behaviour, and thoughts that make humans human.

2   Mead presumably had not come across any female politicians.

5 Abusive

1   The justified replacement of obnoxious and stigmatizing labels, unjustified politically bandwagons, and customary cultural variations, have produced an assortment of terms for genetic, traumatic, or idiopathic damage to brain functioning at or shortly after birth. For example: mental handicap; intellectual disability; intellectual impairment; learning disability; mental retardation; mental sub-normality; feeble-mindedness; and idiocy. None of these terms adequately covers all the problems faced by the people to whom they refer. I have selected 'mental handicap' because it is, arguably, the least-worst option.

7 Insane

1   *Mosi-oa-Tunya* is the name given to Victoria Falls by the Kololo tribe, and translates as the 'Smoke that Thunders'.
2   I am using the terms insanity and madness as synonyms, inclusive of psycho-pathy (which I also take to embrace sociopathy and personality disorder.
3   Not having a photo-copying facility at the time, the version referred to here was obtained via the BBC's internet travel advice service.
4   Diagnostic categories referred to here are from either: (1) *The International Classification of Diseases* (1993) (ICD-10 Classification of Mental and Beha-vioural Disorders Diagnostic Criteria), Geneva: World Health Organization; (2) *The Diagnostic and Statistical Manual of Mental Disorders* (1994) (DSM-IV American Psychiatric Association), Arlington, Virginia: American Psychia-tric Press Association. 'Troublesome-personality-changes disorder' is taken from (1).
5   Sue Pattison (2006) and Sally Hodges (2002) have demonstrated in their respective work on children/young people with learning disabilities and adult with learning disabilities, however, that poor communication need not be a barrier to undergoing therapy.

Conclusion

1   'That's No Way to Say Goodbye', from the CD 'Songs of Leonard Cohen'. Sony Records (1968).
2   'Two Little Hitlers' is the title of a song by Elvis Costello and the Attractions LP Armed Forces (1979; London: Radar).
3   'Walk by me again' is taken from the track 'Dear Heather' on Leonard Cohen's 2004 CD 'Dear Heather' (New York: Columbia Records).

Bibliography

Adler, J. (2006) Freud in our midst, *Newsweek*, 27 March. http://www.msnbc.msn.com/id/11904222/site/newsweek/

American Association for the Advancement of Science (2007) *Science* Medicine/Diseases (archived articles 1995–2007) http://www.sciencemag.org/cgi/collection/medicine

American College of Surgeons (2006) Unnecessary operations http://www.facs.org/fellows_info/statements/stonprin.html#anchor175181

American Counseling Association (2007) Definition of professional counselling. www.http://counseling.org

American Humanist Association (2007) Humanists praise Pete Stark for 'coming out as a nontheist'. http://www.americanhumanist.org/index.html

American Psychological Association (2008) If sex enters into the therapy relationship, Women's Program Office. http://www.apa.org/pi/therapy.html

Asay, T. and Lambert, M. (1999) The empirical case for the common factors in therapy: quantitative findings, in M. Hubble, B. Duncan and S. Miller (eds) *The Heart and Soul of Change: What Works in Therapy*. Washington, DC: American Psychological Association, pp. 33–56.

Association for Psychological Science (2007) *History of APS*. http://www.psycho
logicalscience.org/about/history.cfm

Bacon, F. ([1597] 1985) *Meditationes Sacræ: De Hæresibus* (Religious Meditations,
of Heresies in the Essays). Harmondsworth: Penguin.

Bakan, J. (2004) *The Corporation: The Pathological Pursuit of Profit and Power*.
London: Constable and Robinson.

Banks, T. (2004) The world according to Tony Banks, *The Independent*, 3
February.

Bateman, A. and Fonagy, P. (2004) *Psychotherapy for Borderline Personality Disorder: Mentalization Based Treatment*. Oxford: Oxford University Press.

Bates, Y. (ed.) (2006) *Shouldn't I Be Feeling Better by Now?: Clients' Views of
Therapy*. Basingstoke: Palgrave Macmillan

Baylis, N. (2006) Well-being Institute, University of Cambridge. www.Cambridge
Wellbeing.org

BBC (2002) Botswana immigration: a layman's guide to the requirements of medical
form (accessed 12 November 2007). http://www.bbc.co.uk/dna/hub/A809336.

BBC News (2006) Scientists attack homeopathy move, 25 October. http://news.
bbc.co.uk/1/hi/health/6085242.stm

Beck, U. (1992) *Risk Society: Towards a New Modernity*, trans. M. Ritter. London:
Sage.

Becker, H.S. (1963) *Outsiders: Studies in the Sociology of Deviance*. Glencoe, IL:
Free Press.

Bem, S. and de Jong, H.B. (2006) *Theoretical Issues in Psychology: An Introduction*,
2nd edn. London: Sage.

Bennett, M. (2004) *The Purpose of Counselling and Psychotherapy*. London: Palgrave Macmillan.

Ben-Shahar, T. (2007) *Happier: Finding Pleasure, Meaning and Life's Ultimate
Currency*. Maidenhead: McGraw-Hill.

Benson, O. and Stangroom, J. (2006) *Why Truth Matters*. London: Continuum.

Bentall, R. (1992) A proposal to classify happiness as a psychiatric disorder, *Journal
of Medical Ethics*, 18(20): 94–8.

Bentall, R. (2003) *Madness Explained: Psychosis and Human Nature*. London:
Allen Lane.

Berger, P. and Luckmann, T. (1966) *The Social Construction of Reality: A Treatise
in the Sociology of Knowledge*. London: Allen Lane.

Bhaskar, R. (1998) Philosophy and scientific realism, in M. Archer, R. Bhaskar, A.
Collier, T. Lawson and A. Norrie (eds) *Critical Realism: Essential Readings*.
London: Routledge, pp.16–47.

Blackburn, S. (2006) *Truth: A Guide for the Perplexed*. London: Penguin.

Bocock, R. (1977) *Freud and Modern Society*. London: Van Nostrand Reinhold.

Bond, M. (2003) The pursuit of happiness, *New Scientist Magazine*, 4 October.

Bosely, S. (2006) Doctors urged [by British Medical Association] to be more vigilant
over drugs' side-effects, *The Guardian*, 12 May.

British Association for Counselling and Psychotherapy (2006) *Profile of BACP: Its Structure, Work and Objectives.* http://www.bacp.co.uk

British Humanist Association (2007) 17 Million humanists in Britain! 36% of the population! http://www.humanism.org.uk/site/cms/

Brockman, J. (ed.) (2007) *What is Your Dangerous Idea?: Today's Leading Thinkers on the Unthinkable.* London: Edge/HarperCollins.

Broks, P. (2006) The ego trip, *The Guardian*, 6 May.

Bryson, B. (2003) *A Short History of Nearly Everything.* New York: Bantum.

Buncombe, A. (2004) The defiance of science, *The Independent*, 29 June.

Burkeman, O. (2006) This column will change your life, *The Guardian*, 30 September.

Burton, M. (2004) radical psychology networks: a review and guide, *Journal of Community and Applied Social Psychology*, 14: 119–30.

Burton, R. ([1621] 2001) *The Anatomy of Melancholy.* New York: New York Review of Books.

Buss, D. (2003) *Evolutionary Psychology: The New Science of the Mind.* New York: Allyn and Bacon.

Cameron, D. (2006) Make people happier, says Cameron, BBC News, 22 May. http://news.bbc.co.uk/1/hi/uk_politics/5003314.stm

Carotenuto, A. (1984) *A Secret Symmetry: Sabina Spielrein between Jung and Freud.* London: Routledge and Kegan Paul.

Central Intelligence Agency (2007) *The World Factbook: Zimbabwe.* https://www.cia.gov/library/publications/the-world-factbook/geos/zi.html#Econ

Central Intelligence Agency (2008a) *The World Factbook: Iceland.* https://www.cia.gov/library/publications/the-world-factbook/geos/ic.html

Central Intelligence Agency (2008b) *The World Factbook. Vanuatu.* https://www.cia.gov/library/publications/the-world-factbook/geos/nh.html

Chaplin, J. (1999) *Feminist Counselling in Action.* London: Sage.

Chomsky, N. (2007) *Hegemony or Survival: America's Quest for Global Dominance*, 2nd edn. London: Penguin.

Clark, D.H. (1974) *Social Therapy in Psychiatry.* Harmondsworth: Penguin.

Cockerham, W. (2007) *Social Causes of Health and Disease.* Cambridge: Polity.

Cockerham, W.C. (2005) *Sociology of Mental Disorder*, 7th edn. Upper Saddle River, NJ: Prentice Hall.

Cohen, S. and Taylor, L. (2004) *Escape Attempts: The Theory and Practice of Resistance to Everyday Life*, 2nd edn. London: Routledge.

Collier, P. (2007) *The Bottom Billion: Why the Poorest Countries are Failing and What Can Be Done about It.* Oxford: Oxford University Press.

Collins, B.E. and Raven, B.H. (1969) Group structure: attraction, coalitions, communication and power, in G. Lindzey and E. Aronson (eds) *Handbook of Social Psychology.* Reading, MA: Addison-Wesley.

Comte, A. (1853) *The Positive Philosophy*, trans. M. Martineau. London: Trubner.

Cooper, A. (ed.) (2002) *Sex and the Internet: A Guide Book for Clinicians.* London: Brunner-Routledge.

Cooper, M. et al. (2007) *Handbook for Person-Centred Psychotherapy and Counselling*. Basingstoke: Palgrave.

Crawford, R. (1980) Healthism and the medicalisation of everyday life, *International Journal of Health Services*, 10: 365–88.

Critical Psychology International (2007) About the Network. http://www.criticalpsychology.com/

Crook, S., Pakulski, J. and Waters, M. (1992) *Postmodernization: Change in Advanced Society*. London: Routledge.

Daines, B. (2000) *Psychodynamic Approaches to Sexual Problems*. Buckingham: Open University Press.

Daines, B., Gask, L. and How, A. (2007) *Medical and Psychiatric Issues for Counsellors*, 2nd edn. London: Sage.

Danner, D., Snowdon, D. and Friesen, W. (2001) Positive emotions in early life and longevity: findings from the nun study, *Journal of Personality and Social Psychology*, 80: 804–13.

Darwin, C.R. (1859) *On the Origin of Species by Means of Natural Selection, or the Preservation of Favoured Races in the Struggle for Life*. London: John Murray.

Davies, J., Sandström, S., Shorrocks, A. and Wolff, E. (2006) *The World Distribution of Household Wealth*, December. The World Institute for Development Economics Research of the United Nations University (UNU-WIDER).

de Botton, A. (2006) *The Architecture of Happiness*. London: Hamish Hamilton.

Dellar, R., Curtis, T. and Leslie, E. (eds) (2000) *Mad Pride*. London: Chipmunkapublishing.

Department of Health (2006a) Healthy body, healthier mind: New guidance to improve physical health of mental health patients, Press release, 17 August. http://www.dh.gov.uk/

Department of Health (2006b) Minister announces physical activity role, Press release, 22 August. http://www.dh.gov.uk/

Department of Health (2006c) Further action taken to tackle obesity, Press release, 30 August. http://www.dh.gov.uk/

Derbyshire, D. (2005) Save us from the salt police, say Stilton makers, *Daily Telegraph* 27 December. http://www.telegraph.co.uk

Descartes, R. ([1637] 2007) *Discourse on Method and the Meditations*. New York: Liberal Arts Press.

Diener, R. (2001) Making the best of a bad situation: satisfaction in the slums of Calcutta, *Social Indicators Research*, 55: 329–52.

Doidge, N. (2007) *The Brain That Changes Itself: Stories of Personal Triumph from the Frontiers of Brain Science*. New York: Viking.

Donn, L. (1988) *Freud and Jung: Years of Friendship, Years of Loss*. New York: Collier.

Dryden, W. (2007) *Handbook of Individual Therapy*. London: Sage.

Drysdale, G. (1861) *The Elements of Social Science: Or Physical, Sexual, and Natural Religion*, 4th edn. London: Truelove.

Durkheim, E. ([1897] 1966) *Suicide*. New York: Free Press.

Easterbrook, G. (2004) *The Progress Paradox: How Life Gets Better While People Feel Worse*. New York: Random House.

Economist (2006) Editorial. Happiness and economics: Economics discovers its feelings, *The Economist*, 19 December.

Engels, F. (1999) *The Condition of the Working Class in England*. Oxford: Oxford Paperbacks.

Epstein, W. (2006) *Psychotherapy as Religion: The Civil Divine in America*. Reno, Nevada: University of Nevada.

Esty, A. (2004) The New Wealth of Nations: Does Bhutan have a better way to measure national progress? *American Scientist*, 92(6), November–December. http://www.americanscientist.org

Faris, R. and Dunham, W. (1965) *Mental Disorders in Urban Areas*. Chicago: University of Chicago Press.

Feltham, C. (2007) Ethical agonising, *Therapy Today*, September. http://www.therapytoday.net/archive/current/cover_feature1.html

Feltham, C. and Horton, I. (2005) *The Sage Handbook of Counselling and Psychotherapy*. London: Sage.

Feyerabend, P. (1975) *Against Method: Outline of an Anarchistic Theory of Knowledge*. London: Humanities Press.

Firebaugh, G. and Tach, L. (2005) Money can buy you happiness but only relative to your peer's income, paper presented at the American Sociological Association Centennial Annual Meeting on 14th August, 2005.http://www.asanet.org/page.ww?section=Press&name=Money+Can+Buy+You+Happiness

Fitzpatrick, M. (2000) *The Tyranny of Health: Doctors and the Regulation of Lifestyle*. London: Routledge.

Follain, J. (2007) Analyse this: Freud 'bedded sister-in-law', *The Sunday Times*, 7 January.

Forrester, V. (1999) *The Economic Horror*. Cambridge: Polity.

Foucault, M. (1966) *The Order of Things* (*Les mots et les choses*). Paris: Gallimard.

Foucault, M. (1969) *Archaeology of Knowledge* (*L'Archéologie du Savoir*). London: Routledge.

Foucault, M. (1971) *Madness and Civilisation*. London: Tavistock.

Foucault, M. (1973) *The Birth of the Clinic*. London: Tavistock.

Foucault, M. (1980) *Power/Knowledge, Selected Interviews and Other Writings, 1972–7*. Harvester: Brighton.

Foucault, M. (1985) *The History of Sexuality*. Harmondsworth: Penguin.

Frank, R. (2000) *Luxury Fever*. Princeton, NJ: Princeton University Press.

Frankl, G. (1979/2005) *Failure of the Sexual Revolution*. London: Open Gate.

Frankl, G. (2000) *Foundations of Morality*. London: Open Gate.

Frankl, G. (2003) *The Social History of the Unconscious*. London: Open Gate.

Frankl, G. (2004) *Blueprint for a Sane Society*. London: Open Gate.

Freedheim, D. (ed.) (1992) *History of Psychotherapy: A Century of Change*. Washington, DC: American Psychological Association.

Freidson, E. (1970) *The Profession of Medicine: A Study of the Applied Sociology of Knowledge*. New York: Dodd Mead.

Freidson, E. (1971) *Professional Dominance: The Social Structure of Medical Care*. Chicago: Aldine.

Freidson, E. (1988) *Professional Powers: A Study of the Institutionalization of Formal Knowledge*. Chicago: University of Chicago Press.

Freidson, E. (1994) *Professionalism Reborn: Theory, Prophecy and Policy*. Cambridge: Polity Press.

Freidson, E. (2001) *Professionalism, the Third Logic: On the Practice of Knowledge*. Chicago: University of Chicago Press.

French, J.R.P and Raven, B.H. (1959) The bases of social power, in D. Cartwright (ed.) *Studies in Social Power*. Michigan: University of Michigan Press.

Freud, A. (1936) *Ego and Mechanisms of Defense*, trans. C. Baines. New York: International Universities Press.

Frith, C. (2007) Determining free will, *New Scientist*, 2616, 11 August, 46.

Fromm, E. (1963) *The Sane Society*. London: Routledge and Kegan Paul.

Fugh-Berman, A. (2005) Not in my name: how I was asked to 'author' a ghost-written research paper, *The Guardian*, 21 April.

Fukuyama, F. (1993) *The End of History and the Last Man*. New York: Avon Books.

Fukuyama, F. (2006) *After the Neocons: America at the Crossroads*. London: Profile.

Fuller, S. (1997) *Science*. Buckingham: Open University Press.

Fuller, S. (2007a) *New Frontiers in Science and Technology Studies*. Cambridge: Polity.

Fuller, S. (2007b) *The Knowledge Book: Key Concepts in Philosophy, Science and Culture*. Stocksfield, Northumberland: Acumen.

Fund for Peace (2007) *Failed States Index 2006*. http://www.fundforpeace.org/programs/fsi/fsindex2006.php

Furedi, F. (2003) *Therapy Culture*. London: Routledge.

Gauntlett, D. (2002) *Media, Gender and Identity: An Introduction*. London: Routledge.

Gay, P. (2006) *Freud: A Life for Our Time*, 2nd edn. London: Little Books.

Gergen, K. (1992) *The Saturated Self*. New York: Basic Books.

Giddens, A. (2006) *Sociology*, 5th edn. Cambridge: Polity.

Gilbert, P. (2007) *Psychotherapy and Counselling for Depression*, 3rd edn. London: Sage.

Glyn, A. (2006) *Capitalism Unleashed: Finance, Globalization, and Welfare*. Oxford: Oxford University Press.

Goffman, E. (1959) *The Presentation of Self in Everyday Life*. Harmondsworth: Penguin.

Goffman, E. (1961) *Asylums: Essays on the Social Situation of Mental Patients and Other Inmates*. New York: Doubleday.

Goffman, E. (1963) *Stigma: Notes on the Management of Spoiled Identity*. Harmondsworth: Penguin.

Goldacre, B. (2007a) A new ethics of bullshit, *Guardian*, 23 June. http://www.badscience.net/

Goldacre, B. (2007b) A kind of magic? *Guardian*, 16 November.

Goldacre, B. (2007c) Benefits and risks of homoeopathy, *The Lancet*, 370 (9600): 1672–3.

Goldacre, B. (2008) *Bad Science*. London: Fourth Estate.

Goldman, A. (1999) *Knowledge in a Social World*. Oxford: Clarendon Press.

Goode, E. (2004) Defying psychiatric wisdom – these skeptics say 'prove it', *New York Times*, 9 March. http://www.nytimes.com/

Goodwin, B. (1997) *How the Leopard Changed Its Spots: Evolution of Complexity*. London: Phoenix.

Goodwin, B. (2007) *Nature's Due: Healing Our Fragmented Culture*. Edinburgh: Floris.

Gore, E. (2006) *An Inconvenient Truth: The Planetary Emergency of Global Warming and What We Can Do About It*. London: Bloomsbury.

Gramsci, A. (1971) *Selections from the Prison Notebooks*, trans. and ed Q. Hoare and G.N. Smith. New York: International Publishers.

Greenhalgh, T. and Wessely, S. (2004) 'Health for me': a sociocultural analysis of healthism in the middle classes, *British Medical Bulletin* 69: 197–213 (The British Council).

Greenpeace (2006) Eating up the Amazon. 6 April. http://www.greenpeace.org/raw/content/international/press/reports/eating-up-the-amazon.pdf

Gribbin, J. (2003) *Science: A History, 1534–2001*. London: Penguin.

Gross International Happiness Project (2008) http://www.gross internationalhappiness.org/

Grosskurth, P. (1991) *The Secret Ring: Freud's Inner Circle and the Politics of Psychoanalysis*. London: Jonathan Cape.

Grossman, W. (2006) *The Skeptic*. http://www.skeptic.org.uk/index.php

Habermas, J. (1970) *Towards a Rational Society*. London: Heinemann.

Habermas, J. (1972) *Knowledge and Human Interests*. London: Heinemann.

Habermas, J. (1975) *Legitimation Crisis*, trans. T. McCarthy. Boston: Beacon Press.

Happiness Center (2007) http://www.reflectivehappiness.com

Harding, C. (2001) *Sexuality: Psychoanalytic Perspectives*. London: Brunner-Routledge.

Harley Therapy (2007) Dr Sheri Jacobson. http://www.harleytherapy.co.uk/dr-sheri-jacobson-psychotherapist-and-counsellor.htm

Hart, G. and Wellings, K. (2002) Sexual behaviour and its medicalisation: in sickness and in health, *British Medical Journal*, 324: 896–900.

Harvard Center for Cancer Prevention, Harvard School of Public Health (2007) *Multivitamins: The Basics*. http://hsphsun3.harvard.edu/cancer/risk/multivitamins/basics/index.htm

Hawkes, G. (1991) *A Sociology of Sex and Sexuality*. Buckingham: Open University Press.

Hawkes, G. (1999) *Sex and Pleasure in Western Culture*. Cambridge: Polity.

Hawking, S. (1995) *A Brief History of Time: From the Big Bang to Black Holes*. New York: Bantam.

Hazelton, M. and Morrall, P. (2008) Mental health, the law, and human rights, in P. Barker (ed.) *Psychiatric and Mental Health Nursing: The Craft of Caring*. London: Hodder Arnold, Chapter 70.

Hedges, F. (2005) *An Introduction to Systemic Therapy with Individuals: A Social Constructionist Approach*. London: Palgrave Macmillan.

Hind, J. (2007) Nervous free will, *New Scientist*, 2619: 24.

Hobbes, T. ([1651] 1998) *Leviathan*. Oxford: Oxford University Press.

Hodges, S. (2002) *Counselling Adults with Learning Disabilities*. Basingstoke: Palgrave Macmillan.

Holmes, B., Kleiner, K., Douglas, K. and Bond, M. (2003) Reasons to be cheerful, *New Scientist Magazine*, 4 October, 2415.

Holmes, J. (2002) All you need is cognitive behaviour therapy? *British Medical Journal*, 324: 288–94.

Holzman, L. and Mendez, R. (eds) (2003) *Psychological Investigations: A Clinician's Guide to Social Therapy*. New York: Guildford.

House, R. (2003) *Therapy Beyond Modernity: Deconstructing and Transcending Profession-Centred Therapy*. London: Karnac.

Hoxter, H. (1999) *The Nature and Scope of Counselling*. http://www.educ.sfu.ca/iac/ORIGIN.HTML (accessed 27 February 2007).

Hudson-Allez, G. (2005) *Sex and Sexuality: Questions and Answers for Counsellors and Therapists*. London: Whurr.

Illich, I. (1975) *Medical Nemesis: The Expropriation of Health*. London: Marian Boyars.

Illich, I., Zola, I. and McKnight, J. (1977) *Disabling Professions*. London: Marion Boyars.

Independent Practitioners Network (2007) Personal communication by email.

International Association for Counselling (2007) Affiliated organisations. http://www.iac-irtac.org/organisations/

International Institute for Strategic Studies (2008) Armed Conflict Data Base. http://www.iiss.org/publications/armed-conflict-database/

International Psychoanalytical Association (2007) *The Origin and Development of the IPA*. http://www.ipa.org.uk

Ironside, V. (2006) Anti-therapy, in Y. Bates (ed.) *Shouldn't I Be Feeling Better by Now?: Clients' Views of Therapy*. Basingstoke: Palgrave Macmillan, pp. 114–22.

James, O. (2007) *Affluenza*. London: Vermillion.

Jarrett, C. (2008) When therapy causes harm, *The Psychologist*, 21(1): 10–12.

Jeffers, S. (2007) *Feel the Fear and Do It Anyway*. London: Random House.

Jha, A. (2007) From arthritis to diabetes: scientists unlock genetic secrets of diseases afflicting millions, *The Guardian*, 7 June.

Johnstone, L. (2000) *Users and Abusers of Psychiatry: A Critical Look at Psychiatric Practice*. London: Brunner-Routledge.

Jung, C. (1966) *The Collected Works of C. G. Jung*. Princeton, NJ: Princeton University Press.

Klein, N. (2007) *The Shock Doctrine: The Rise of Disaster Capitalism*. London: Allen Lane.

Klobert, E. (2006) *Field Notes from a Catastrophe: Climate Change – Is Time Running Out?* London: Bloomsbury.

Kuhn, T. (1962) *The Structure of Scientific Revolutions*. Chicago: University of Chicago Press.

Lacquer, T. (1990) *Making Sex: Body and Gender from the Greeks to Freud*. Cambridge, MA: Harvard University Press.

Lacquer, T. (2003) *Solitary Sex: A Cultural History of Masturbation*. New York: Zone.

Laing, R.D. (1965) *The Divided Self*. Harmondsworth: Pelican.

Laing, R,D. and Esterson, A. (1964) *Sanity, Madness and the Family*. London: Harmondsworth: Penguin.

Layard, R. (2006a) *The Depression Report: A New Deal for Depression and Anxiety Disorders*. The London School of Economics Centre for Economic Performance's Mental Health Policy Group. London: London School of Economics.

Layard, R. (2006b) *Happiness: Lessons from a New Science*. London: Penguin.

Leader, D. (2007) A dark age for mental health, *The Guardian*, 13 October.

Leader, D. and Corfield, D. (2007) *Why Do People Get Ill?* London: Hamish Hamilton.

LeBon, T. (2001) *Wise Therapy: Philosophy for Counsellors*. London: Sage.

Legrain, P. (2003) *Open World: The Truth about Globalisation*. London: Abacus.

Legrain, P. (2006) Globalisation is working, *Prospect Magazine*, Issue 125, August. http://www.philippelegrain.com/legrain/2006/07/globalisation

Leigh, A. and Wolfers, J. (2006) *Happiness and the Human Development Index: Australia is Not a Paradox*. National Bureau of Economic Research Working Paper No. 11925. http://www.nber.org/papers/w11925

Lemert, E.M. (1951) *Social Pathology: A Systematic Approach to the Study of Sociopathic Behavior*. New York: McGraw-Hill.

Lilienfeld, S., Lynn, S. and Lohr, J. (eds) (2004) *Science and Pseudoscience in Clinical Psychology*. New York: Guilford.

Lilienfeld, S. and O'Donohue, W. (eds) (2008) *The Great Ideas of Clinical Science: 17 Principles That Every Mental Health Professional Should Understand*. London: Routledge.

Lilienfeld, S., Ruscio, J. and Lynn, S. (eds) (2009) *Navigating the Mindfield: A Guide to Separating Science from Pseudoscience in Mental Health*. New York: Prometheus.

Lindberg, C. (1992) *The Beginnings of Western Science: The European Scientific Tradition in Philosophical, Religious, and Institutional Context, 600 B.C. to A.D. 1450*. Chicago: University of Chicago Press.

Lodge, D. (1995) *Therapy*. Harmondsworth: Penguin.

Lovelock, J. (2006) *The Revenge of Gaia: Why the Earth Is Fighting Back – and How We Can Still Save Humanity*. London: Allen Lane.

Maines, R. (1999) *The Technology of Orgasm: 'Hysteria,' the Vibrator, and Women's Sexual Satisfaction*. Baltimore, MD: The Johns Hopkins University Press.

Malhotra, V.A. (1987) Habermas' sociological theory as a basis for clinical practice with small groups, *Clinical Sociology Review*, 5, 181–92.

Mann, D. (1997) *Psychotherapy: An Erotic Relationship – Transference and Countertransference, Passions*. London: Routledge.

Marx, K. ([1843] 1970) *Critique of Hegel's Philosophy of Right*. Cambridge: Cambridge University Press.

Marx, K. ([1844] 1959) *Economic and Philosophical Manuscripts of 1844*, trans. M. Milligan and ed. D. Struik. London: Lawrence and Wishart.

Marx, K. ([1867] 1971) *Das Kapital/Capital: A Critique of Political Economy*, ed. F. Engels. London: Lawrence and Wishart.

Masson, J. (1990) *Against Therapy*. London: Fontana.

Mathiason, N. and Aglionby, J. (2006) Exposed: life at factory that supplies our fashion stores (Prek Seer, Cambodia), *The Observer*, 23 April.

McCarthy, P., Walker, J. and Rain, J. (1998) *Telling It As It Is: The Client Experience of Relate Counselling*. Newcastle-upon-Tyne: Newcastle Centre for Family Studies.

McGuire, W. (ed.) (1974) *The Freud/Jung Letters: The Correspondence between Sigmund Freud and C. G. Jung*. Princeton, NJ: Princeton University Press.

McKeown, K., Lehane, P., Rock, R., Haase, T. and Pratschke, J. (2002) *Unhappy Marriages: Does Counselling Help?* Maynooth, Co. Kildare, Ireland: ACCORD Catholic Marriage Care Service and Department of Social and Family Affairs in Ireland.

McLeod, J. (2003) *An Introduction to Counselling*, 3rd edn. Maidenhead: Open University Press.

McLuhan, M. (1964) *Understanding Media: The Extensions of Man*. New York: McGraw-Hill.

McNamee, S. and Gergen, K. (eds) (1992) *Therapy as Social Construction*. London: Sage.

McQuail, D. (2005) *McQuail's Mass Communication Theory*, 5th edn. London: Sage.

McTaggart, L. (2005) *What Doctors Don't Tell You: The Truth About the Dangers of Modern Medicine*, 2nd edn. London: Thorsons.

Mead, G.H. (1934) *Mind, Self, and Society*. Chicago: University of Chicago Press.

Merton, R.K. (1938) Social structure and anomie, *American Sociological Review*, 3 (October), 672–82.

Merton, R.K. (1957) *Social Theory and Social Structure*. Glencoe, IL: The Free Press.

Mill, J.S. ([1861] 2001) *Utilitarianism*, ed. G. Sher, 2nd edn. Indianapolis, IN: Hackett.

Miller, P. and Rose, N. (1986) *The Power of Psychiatry*. Cambridge: Polity.

Mills, C.W. (1959) *The Sociological Imagination*. Oxford: Oxford University Press.

Mirkin, M. (ed.) (1994) *Women in Context: Toward a Feminist Reconstruction of Psychotherapy*. New York: Guilford Press.

Mirza, S.K. (2002) Why critical scrutiny of Islam is an utmost necessity, *Islam Watch*, 23 May.

Monbiot, G. (2004) *The Age of Consent*. New York: Harper Perennial.

Monbiot, G. (2007) *Heat: How We Can Stop the Planet Burning*. London: Penguin.

Monet, V. (2005) Escorts as therapists. http//:www.VeronicaMonet.com accessed January 2007.

Morrall, P. (2000) *Madness and Murder*. London: Whurr.

Morrall, P. (2001) *Sociology and Nursing*. London: Routledge.

Morrall, P. (2006a) *Murder and Society*. Chichester: John Wiley & Sons, Ltd.

Morrall, P. (2006b) Psychiatry and psychiatric nursing in the new world order, in J. Cutcliffe and M. Ward (eds) *Key Debates in Psychiatric and Mental Health Care*. Oxford: Elsevier.

Morrall, P. (2007a) Murder and society: why commit murder? *Criminal Justice Matters*, 66.

Morrall, P (2007b) The trouble with therapy. *Irish Association for Counselling and Psychotherapy*, 7(3): 14–18.

Morrall, P. (2008) Snake oil peddling: complementary and alternative medicine and the occupational status of doctors and nurses, in J. Adams and P. Tovey (eds) *Complementary and Alternative Medicine in Nursing and Midwifery: Towards a Critical Social Science*. London: Routledge.

Morrall, P. and Hazelton, M. (2004) *Mental Health: Global Policies and Human Rights*. Chichester: Wiley.

Museo, Larco (2007) Aztec eroticism in ceramics: Lima, Peru: Museo Larco. http://museolarco.perucultural.org.pe/iindex.html

Neal, C. (2000) *Issues in Therapy with Lesbian, Gay, Bisexual and Transgender Clients*. Buckingham: Open University Press.

Nelson-Jones, R. (2005) *Theory and Practice of Counselling and Therapy*. London: Sage.

Nettle, D. (2005) *Happiness: The Science Behind Your Smile*. Oxford: Oxford University Press.

Newman, F. and Holzman, L. (2000) The relevance of Marx to therapeutics in the 21st century, *New Therapist*, 5: 24–7.

NHS Direct Online Health Encyclopedia (2007) Health encyclopaedia. http://www.nhsdirect.nhs.uk/encyclopaedia/

O'Hara, M. (1995) Carl Rogers: scientist and mystic, *Journal of Humanistic Psychology*, 35(4): 40–53.

Office for National Statistics (2005) http://www.statistics.gov.uk/methods_quality/ns_sec/default.asp (accessed September 2006).

Parsons, T. (1951) *The Social System*. London: Routledge and Kegan Paul.

Patterson, R. and Weijer, C. (1998) D'oh! An analysis of the medical care provided to the family of Homer J. Simpson, *Canadian Medical Association Journal*, 159(12): 1480–1.

Pattison, S. (2006) Making every child matter: a model for good practice in counselling children and young people with learning disabilities, *Pastoral Care in Education*, 24(2), 22–8.

Perkin, H. (2000) Exploring professional values for the 21st century: crisis in the professions – ambiguities, origins and current problems. The Royal Society for the Encouragement of Arts, Manufactures & Commerce. http://www.thersa.org.uk/acrobat/Perkin1.pdf

Perrons, D. (2004) *Globalisation and Social Change: People and Places in a Divided World*. London: Routledge.

Picard, L. (2006) *Victorian London: The Life of a City 1840–1870*. London: Orion.

Pilger, J. (2007) *War on Democracy*. Lionsgate Films. http://www.lionsgatefilms.com

Pilgrim, D. (1997) *Psychotherapy and Society*. London: Sage.

Pilgrim, D. and Rogers, A. (2002) *Mental Health and Inequality*. Basingstoke: Palgrave Macmillan.

Pinker, S. (2003) *The Blank Slate: The Modern Denial of Human Nature*. London: Penguin.

Polivy, J. (2001) The false hope syndrome: unrealistic expectations of self-change, *International Journal of Obesity and Related Metabolic Disorders*, 25(1), supplement, pp. 80–4.

Pope, W. (1976) *Durkheim's Suicide: A Classic Analyzed*. Chicago: University of Chicago Press.

Porter, R. (2003) *Blood and Guts: A Short History of Medicine*. London: Penguin.

Priebe, S. and Wright, D. (2006) The provision of psychotherapy – an international comparison, *The Journal of Public Mental Health*, 5(3): 12–22.

Pritz, A. (ed.) (2002) *Globalized Psychotherapy*. Vienna: Facultas Universitätsverlag.

Proctor, G., Cooper, M., Sanders, P. and Malcolm, B. (2006) *Politicizing the Person-Centred Approach*. Ross-on-Wye, Hereford: PCC.

PsychOz (2007) *Resources for Effective Psychotherapy and Counselling*. http://www.psychotherapy.com.au/

Public Library of Science Medicine (2006) 34. http://medicine.plosjournals.org

Purkey, W. and Schmidt, J. (1995) *Invitational Counseling: A Self Concept Approach to Professional Practice*. Pacific Grove, CA: Brooks Cole.

Racevskis, K. (ed.) (1999) *Critical Essays on Michel Foucault*. New York: G.K. Hall.

Radical Psychology Network (2007) *The Radical Psychology Network*. http://www.radpsynet.org/

Redelmeier, D. and Kahneman, D. (1996) Patients' memories of painful medical treatments: real time and retrospective evaluations of two minimally invasive procedures, *Pain*, 66(1): 3–8.

Redelmeier, D., Katz, J. and Kahneman, D. (2003) Memories of colonoscopy: a randomized trial, *Pain*, 104(1–2): 187–94.

Reich, W. (1989) *Function of the Orgasm*. London: Souvenir.

Relate (2006a) Leading voluntary sector agency is set to open a pioneering training centre for couple, Press release, 21 June. http://www.relate.org.uk/media centre/pressreleases/PressRelease

Relate (2006b) Relate, the Relationship People. http://www.relate.org.uk/ (accessed 12 September 2006).

Relate (2007) Research and statistics. http://www.relate.org.uk/aboutus/research andstatistics/

Relate (2008) Relate, the relationship people. We're here to help you find the answers. http://www.relate.org.uk/

Rice, M. (2006) Editorial, *Psychologies Magazine*. September, 1, http://www. psychologies.co.uk/expert_home.php

Ritzer, G. (2006) *Contemporary Sociological Theory and its Classic Roots: The Basics*, 2nd edn. New York: McGraw-Hill.

Roehr, B. (2006) Institute of Medicine report strives to reduce medication errors, *BMJ*, 333, p.220 (29 July), doi:10.1136/bmj.333.7561.220-f

Rogers, C. (1951) *Client Centred Therapy*. London: Constable.

Rohen, D. (2006) Global trade in sex toys, *Counterpunch*, 2/3 December. http:// www.counterpunch.org

Rose, N. (1985) *The Psychological Complex: Psychology, Politics and Society in England 1869–1939*. London: Routledge and Kegan Paul.

Rose, N. (1990) *Governing the Soul: The Shaping of the Private Self*, 2nd edn. London: Free Association Books.

Rose, N. (2000) Government and control, *British Journal of Criminology*, 40(2): 321–39.

Rose, N. (2007) Power and subjectivity: critical history and psychology. (Academy for the Study of the Psychoanalytic Arts.) http://www.academyanalyticarts.org/ rose1.htm

Rose, S. (1997) *Lifelines: Biology, Freedom, Determinism*. Harmondsworth: Penguin.

Roth, A. and Fonagy, P. (2006) *What Works for Whom: A Critical Review of Psychotherapy Research*, 2nd edn. London: Guilford.

Rowling, J.K. (1997) *Harry Potter and the Philosopher's Stone*. London: Bloomsbury.

Russell, B. (1961) *History of Western Civilisation*. London: Routledge.

Russell, J. (1993) *Out of Bounds: Sexual Exploitation in Counselling and Therapy*. London: Sage.

Samuels, A. (2006) Politics on the couch? Psychotherapy and society: some possibilities and some limitations, in N. Totton (ed.) *The Politics of Psychotherapy: New Perspectives.* Maidenhead: Open University Press.

Sandford, A. (2007) Strike fever spreading in France. BBC News. http://news.bbc.co.uk/1/hi/world/europe/7102840.stm

Sartre, J. ([1938] 1965) *Nausea (La Nausée).* Harmondsworth: Penguin.

Schaler, J. (1995) Good therapy also draws comparisons between psychotherapy and prostitution, *The Interpsych Newsletter*, August–September 2(7). http://www.schaler.net/fifth/cultbusting.html

Scheff, T.J. (1966) *Being Mentally Ill: A Sociological Theory.* Chicago: Aldine.

Schultz, T. (2001) Distance communication, *Für Soziologie*, 30(2): 85–102.

Schumaker, J.F. (2006) The happiness conspiracy: What does it mean to be happy in a modern consumer society? http://www.newint.org/columns/essays/2006/07/01/happiness-conspiracy

Scull, A.T. (1984) *Decarceration: Community Treatment and the Deviant – a Radical View*, 2nd edn. Cambridge: Polity Press.

Scull, A.T. (1992) *Social Order – Mental Disorder: Anglo-American Psychiatry in Historical Perspective.* Berkeley, CA: University of California Press.

Scull, A.T. (1993) *The Most Solitary of Afflictions: Madness and Society in Britain, 1700–1900.* New Haven, CT: Yale University Press.

Select Committee on Science and Technology (2006) *Scientific Advice, Risk and Evidence Based Policy Making.* No. 63 of Session 2005–06 8 November. http://www.parliament.uk/parliamentary_committees/science_and_technology_committee/scitech081106.cfm

Seligman, M. (2003) *Authentic Happiness: Using the New Positive Psychology to Realise Your Potential for Lasting Fulfilment.* London: Nicholas Brealey.

Seligman, M. (2006) *Learned Optimism: How to Change Your Mind and Your Life.* New York: Vintage.

Seligman, M. (2007) http://www.authentichappiness.sas.upenn.edu

Sense About Science (2006) Statement on Evidence-Based Medicine and The Medicines for Human Use (National Rules for Homeopathic Products) Regulations 2006. http://www.senseaboutscience.org.uk/

Seu, B. and Heenan, C. (eds) (1998) *Feminism and Psychotherapy: Reflections on Contemporary Theories and Practices.* London: Sage.

Shiva, V. (2000) BBC Reith Lecture 2000 Poverty and Globalisation. http://news.bbc.co.uk/hi/english/static/events/reith_2000/lecture5.stm

Shorter, E. (1997) *A History of Psychiatry.* New York: Wiley.

Singer, M. and Lalich, J. (2002) *Crazy Therapies : What Are They? Do They Work?* Chichester: Jossey-Bass Wiley.

Smail, D. (1999) Psychotherapy, society and the individual, talk given at the 'Ways with Words' festival of literature, Dartington, 12 July 1999. http://www.djsmail.com/

Smail, D. (2001) *Psychology and Power: Understanding Human Action.* http://www.davidsmail.freeuk.com

Smail, D. (2002) Psychology and power: understanding human action, *The Journal of Critical Psychology, Counselling and Psychotherapy*, 2: 1–10.

Smail, D. (2006) Truth, politics and psychological therapy – may the lord deliver us from professional uncertainty, talk given to the Humanities and Mental Health Research Network in Nottingham, 1 March 2006. http://www.djsmail.com/

Smith, R. (2002) Book review of *Limits to Medicine. Medical Nemesis: The Expropriation of Health* by Ivan Illich, *BMJ* (13 April) 324: 923.

Smith, R. and Moynihan, R. (2002) Too much medicine? Almost certainly, *BMJ* 13 April, 324: 859–60.

Snyder, C. and Lopez, S. (eds) (2004) *Handbook of Positive Psychology*. Oxford: Oxford University Press.

Spinelli, E. (1994) *Demystifying Therapy*. London: Constable.

Storr, A. (2001) *Freud: A Very Short Introduction*. Oxford: Oxford University Press.

Strate, L., Jacobson, R. and Gibson, S. (eds) (2002) *Communication and Cyberspace: Social Interaction in an Electronic Environment*. Creskill, NJ: Hampton Press.

Sufi Psychology Association (2007) Sufi Psychotherapy: Healing the Soul. http://www.sufipsychology.org/

Sweatshop Watch (2006) Modern day sweatshops. http://www.sweatshop watch.org/

Szasz, T. (1972) *The Myth of Mental Illness*. St Albans: Paladin.

Szasz, T. (1974) *The Myth of Mental Illness: Foundations for a Theory of Personal Conduct*, rev. edn. New York: Harper and Row.

Szasz, T. (1978) *Myth of Psychotherapy: Mental Healing as Religion, Rhetoric and Repression*. London: Doubleday.

Szasz, T. (1993) Curing, coercing, and claims-making: a reply to critics, *British Journal of Psychiatry*, 162: 797–800.

Szasz, T. and Hollender, M.H. (1956) A contribution to the philosophy of medicine: the basic models of the doctor–patient relationship, *Archives of Internal Medicine*, 97: 585–92.

Tallis, F. (2005) *Love Sick*. London: Arrow Books.

Tarot UK (2006) Welcome. Tarot UK offers you information on tarot, tarot readings, psychic readings and matters of spirituality. http://www.tarotuk.co.uk/

Tarot.com (2006) What do your past lives reveal? http://www.tarot.com/tarot/index.php

Templar, R. (2005) *The Rules of Life: A Personal Code for Living a Better, Happier, More Successful Kind of Life*. London: Pearson.

Thagard, P. (2005) *Mind: Introduction to Cognitive Science*, 2nd edn. Cambridge, MA: MIT Press.

The American Psychotherapy Association (2007) About the American Psychotherapy Association Mission Statement. http://www.americanpsychotherapy.com/about.php

The British Psychoanalytic Council (2007) About the British Psychoanalytic Council http://www.bcp.org.uk/about.html

The Future Foundation (2004) *The Age of Therapy*. London: The Future Foundation.

The Happy Planet Index (2006) Economics as if people and the planet mattered: Friends of the Earth. http://www.neweconomics.org/gen/uploads/ dl44k145g5scuy453044gqbu11072006194758.pdf

The Psychotherapy and Counselling Federation of Australia (2007) Definition of Psychotherapy and Counselling. http://www.pacfa.org.au

Thomas, B. and Dorling, D. (2007) *Identity in Britain: A Cradle-to-Grave Atlas*. Bristol: University of Bristol Policy Press.

Totton, N. (2000) *Psychotherapy and Politics*. London: Sage.

Totton, N. (ed.) (2006) *The Politics of Psychotherapy: New Perspectives*. Maidenhead: Open University Press.

Turkle, S. (2005) *The Second Self: Computers and the Human Spirit*, 2nd edn. Cambridge, MA: MIT Press.

United Kingdom Council for Psychotherapy (2007) *What Is the Difference between Counselling and Psychotherapy?* http://www.psychotherapy.org.uk/

United Nations (2006) *Social Indicators*. United Nations Statistical Division. http:// unstats.un.org/unsd/demographic/products/socind/health.htm

United Nations (2007) Global unemployment remains at historic high despite strong economic growth. United Nations News Centre. http://www.un.org/apps/ news/story.asp?NewsID=21335&Cr=unemployment&Cr1

United Nations (2008a) *Agenda*. http://www.un.org/issues/

United Nations (2008b) *United Nations Peacekeeping Operations*. http://www.un. org/Depts/dpko/dpko/pub/year_review06/PKmissions.pdf

Ward, D. (2006) School spreads a little happiness with lessons on how to cheer up. *The Guardian*, 18 April.

Weber, M. (1948) *From Max Weber: Essays in Sociology*, trans. and ed. H.H. Gerth and C.W. Mills. London: Routledge and Kegan Paul.

Webster, R. (2005) *Why Freud Was Wrong: Sin, Science and Psychoanalysis*, 3rd edn. Oxford: Orwell Press.

Wheen, F. (2000) *Karl Marx*. London: Fourth Estate.

Wheen, F. (2005) Why Marx is man of the moment. *The Observer*, 17 July.

Wilkinson, G., McKenzie, K. and Harpham, T. (eds) (2005) *Social Capital and Mental Health*. London: Jessica Kingsley.

Wilkinson, I. (2005) *Suffering: A Sociological Introduction*. Cambridge: Polity.

Williams, H. (2006) *Britain's Power Elites: The Rebirth of a Ruling Class*. London: Constable and Robinson.

Williams, P. (2003) The potential perils of personal issues in coaching, *International Coaching in Organizations*, 2: 21–30.

Williams, R. (2004) Christmas message from the Archbishop of Canterbury to the Anglican Communion, Press release, 17 November. http://www.archbishop ofcanterbury.org

Wintour, P. (2006) Blair plans new social contract: agreements between individuals and state on health, schools and police, *The Guardian*, 24 November.

Wollaston, S. (2007) Sleep badly last night? *The Guardian*, 20 February.

Wolpert, L. (2005) The sceptical inquirer. *The Independent*, 9 February.

Woolfe, R. et al. (2003) *Handbook of Counselling Psychology*. London: Sage.

World Council for Psychotherapy (2007) http://www.worldpsyche.org/

World Health Organization (2005) World Health Organization partners with Joint Commission and Joint Commission International to eliminate medical errors worldwide. http://www.jointcommission.org/NewsRoom/PressKits/WHO/nr_082305.htm

World Health Organization (2008) Mental health: the bare facts. http://www.who.int/mental_health

World Institute for Development Economics Research (2006) *The World Distribution of Household Wealth, December 2006*. Helsinki: United Nations University.

World Revolution (2008) The State of the World. http://www.worldrevolution.org/

Wosket, V. (2006) *Egan's Skilled Helper Model*. London: Routledge.

Yergin, D. and Stanislaw, J. (1998) *The Commanding Heights: The New Reality of Economic Power*. New York: Simon and Schuster.

Young-Bruehl, E. (1990) *Freud on Women*. London: Hogarth.

Index

COUNSELLING SKILL

John McLeod

'Many books have been written on "counselling skills" to complement a counselling skills training course. The difference between this book and those based on counselling skills is that it provides a less daunting, more user-friendly approach to talking and listening to people...Counselling Skill is a refreshing read that has aided my continuing professional development through a process of self-reflection. It has also influenced my approach as a nurse now that I have applied counselling skill concepts during social interactions with patients'

Nursing Standard

- Does your job involve working with people?
- Do you know what to do when your clients or colleagues want to talk to you about difficult issues in their lives?
- Would you like to improve your ability to listen and help others?

This book is written for practitioners such as teachers, doctors, community workers, nurses and social workers, whose counselling role is embedded within other work functions. A framework is introduced, that allows the reader to draw on knowledge and competencies from their own personal and professional experience, as well as from a range of approaches to counselling, that will help them to help others.

The majority of people who seek help for personal issues do not consult specialist counsellors or psychotherapists, but instead look for support from people who are close to hand. In many instances, the counselling conversations that they have may last for no more than a few minutes. This book equips readers with methods and strategies for working effectively in such circumstances.

Counselling Skill outlines the abilities needed for counselling others – listening carefully, self-awareness, instillation of hope, being reliable and trustworthy, a capacity to engage with emotion – and suggests how these everyday skills may be used to help others to help themselves. In order to help those new to the ideas in the book, each chapter is supported by examples, as well as evidence from research studies.

This book is key reading for people working in helping, managing or supervisory roles: it provides efficient and ethical strategies that will improve their ability to assist or advise others. It is also of use to counsellors and counselling students who wish to develop a better understanding of their craft.

Contents: *Preface – Introduction – Defining counselling – Basic principles of embedded counselling – The counselling menu: goals, tasks and methods – Setting the scene: Preparation for offering a counselling relationship – Making a space to meet – Working collaboratively: building a relationship – Having a useful conversation: "Just talking" – Resolving difficult feelings and emotions – Learning to do something different: Working together to change behaviour – Dealing with difficult situations in counselling – Putting it all together: Doing good work – References – Index.*

2007 288pp
978-0-335-21809-7 (Paperback) 978-0-335-21810-3 (Hardback)

AN INTRODUCTION TO COUNSELLING
Third Edition

John McLeod

Reviews of the second edition:

'It is impossible to do justice to such an exhaustive, broadbased and very readable work in a short review. Professor McLeod has been meticulous, and with true scientific impartiality has looked at, studied and described the many strands and different schools of thought and methods that can lead towards successful counselling.'

Therapy Weekly

'This is a fascinating, informative, comprehensive and very readable book...McLeod has produced a text that offers a great deal no matter what your level of competence or knowledge.'

Journal of Interprofessional Care

'...one of the book's strengths is McLeod's willingness to go beyond a history of the development of counselling or a beginner's technical manual...{and to} consider the political dimensions of counselling and the relevance of power to counselling relationships. A worthwhile acquisition for therapeutic community members, whatever their discipline or background.'

Therapeutic Communities

This thoroughly revised and expanded version of the bestselling text, *An Introduction to Counselling*, provides a comprehensive introduction to the theory and practice of counselling and therapy. It is written in a clear, accessible style, covers all the core approaches to counselling, and takes a critical, questioning approach to issues of professional practise. Placing each counselling approach in its social and historical context, the book also introduces a wide range of contemporary approaches, including narrative therapy, systemic, feminist and multicultural.

This third edition includes a new chapter on the important emerging approach of philosophical counselling, and a chapter on the counselling relationship, as well as expanded coverage of attachment theory, counselling on the internet, and solution-focused therapy. The text has been updated throughout, with additional illustrative vignettes and case studies.

Current, comprehensive and readable, with exhaustive references, An Introduction to Counselling is a classic introduction to its subject.

Contents: Preface – An introduction to counselling – The cultural and historical origins of counselling – Counselling theories: Diversity and convergence – Themes and issues in the psychodynamic approach to counselling – From behaviourism to constructivism: The cognitive-behavioural approach to counselling – Theory and practice of the person-centred approach – Working with systems – Feminist approaches: the radicalization of counselling – Narrative approaches to counselling: Working with stories – Multiculturalism as an approach to counselling – Philosophical counselling – The counselling relationship – The process of counselling – The politics of counselling: Empowerment, control and difference – Morals, values and ethics in counselling practice – The organizational context of counselling – Alternative modes of delivery – The role of research in counselling and therapy – The skills and qualities of the effective counsellor – Training and supervision in counselling – Beyond an introduction: Continuing the conversation – References – Index.

2003 640pp
978-0-335-21189-0 (Paperback)

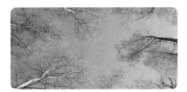
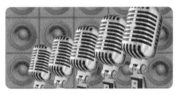
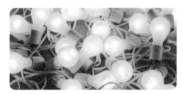
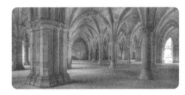
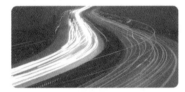
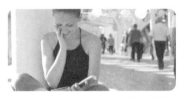
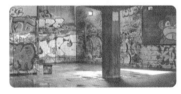